COACHES' GUIDE TO NUTRITION AND WEIGHT CONTROL

Coaches' Guide to
NUTRITION
& Weight Control

Patricia Eisenman
Associate Professor
Director of the Human
Performance Laboratory
Marshall University

Dennis A. Johnson
Head Wrestling Coach
Sheffield Area High School
Sheffield, Pennsylvania

Human Kinetics Publishers

Champaign, Illinois

Publications Director
Richard D. Howell

Copy Editor
Margery Brandfon

Typesetter
Sandra Meier

Text Design and Layout
Denise Peters

Cover Design and Layout
Jack W. Davis

Library of Congress Catalog Number: 81-82452

ISBN: 0-931250-25-0

9 8 7 6 5 4 3 2 1

Human Kinetics Publishers, Inc.
Box 5076
Champaign, Illinois 61820

2-18-83

Acknowledgments

There are a host of people whose help we would like to acknowledge. Rainer Martens and Margery Brandfon, from Human Kinetics, read and reread while Pat Mulcahy and Patty Perdue, our typists, typed and retyped.

Gary Lapelle's illustrations did a super job of capturing the agony as well as the ecstasy of weight control. The weight training photographs were due to the patience of Jim Arnold and the willingness of Beth Hooker and Bruce Kowalski to squeeze the photographic sessions in between swimming practices.

Finally, we'd like to thank our students and athletes who, over the years, have provided valuable feedback and encouragement.

Contents

Preface

These are exciting times to be involved in sport. Not only are millions and millions of people participating in sport, but many of these athletes and their coaches are becoming interested in the scientific aspects of their sports. For years, Americans have embraced science and technology in the home and workplace, but only recently has science entered the locker room. Coaches today not only want to learn about the latest technique or strategy, but they want to know about sport physiology, biomechanics, and sport psychology as well. They have such questions about nutrition and weight control as: Can protein supplements really build muscle? Should we give Vitamin C tablets to our athletes? There are no one-sentence answers to these questions. Rather, the best answers we have at this time lie in understanding body composition and how it is related to physical performance; understanding ideal body weight and how it can be attained; and understanding how to fuel the body for sport.

This knowledge and much more regarding nutrition and weight control is presented in this book. We have gathered the most accurate information possible from the sport scientist about weight control, muscle fueling, and hydration. We will describe step-by-step procedures so you can determine the *ideal weight* for each of your athletes. Then we will tell you precisely how to help your athletes achieve that weight.

We have tried to bridge the proverbial gap between research and practice, by examining both the "why" and "how" of nutrition and weight control. You will see the importance of using this information on a day-to-day basis as you coach. So this book is not the type that you can read once and then put away. We encourage you to read it and then use it as a reference when you need information. In this way, you can help your athletes condition themselves for more successful participation as well as help them formulate sound nutritional habits. Nothing would make us happier than for this book to help you do so.

Patricia A. Eisenman, PhD
Dennis Johnson

Foreword

All athletes, regardless of their sport, their age, or their sex, perform best at a specific weight. This optimum competitive weight varies from athlete to athlete and changes as individuals grow and develop in their sport.

To know how to determine this weight and, more importantly, how to safely attain it, has been the best kept secret since Paris of Troy discovered Achilles' weak point. Now, *Coaches' Guide to Nutrition and Weight Control* finally reveals this secret. It provides the coach, parent, administrator, and athlete with clear, precise, basic knowledge on finding—and performing at—optimum weight.

This book invites your reading! It's a must for everyone concerned about teaching and training the "total" athlete.

Steve Combs, Executive Director
United States
Wrestling Federation

Chapter 1

Weight Control and Energy Management

To most Americans, weight control conjures up images of the "Battle of the Bulge"—of middle-aged women donning jogging togs to venture out to the local neighborhood health salon, and of pot-bellied men exercising to regain the belt size of years gone by. Weight control, for the average person means watching the dial drop—or at least not go up—on the bathroom scale.

Weight control in sport, however, means much more than fluctuations on the bathroom scale. It means athletes striving to achieve their *ideal weight* for optimal performance. Ideal weight is just the right combination of muscle, bone, and fat so that the athletes have sufficient size, strength, and energy to meet the demands of their sport without any excess fat.

To attain their ideal weight, athletes may need to either lose *or* gain weight, depending on the athlete and sport being played. Or, athletes may be at the proper weight, but need to change the proportion of muscle and fat. In chapter 2, you will learn how to measure ideal weight, and in subsequent chapters, you will learn energy man-

1

agement procedures, which you can use to help athletes lose or gain weight safely and effectively. In addition, we will tell you how to feed your athletes with energy-packed, high octane fuel.

In the competitive world of sport, coaches can no longer afford to use the time-honored binocular scanning method, better known as the "eyeball" technique, for determining whether an athlete should lose or gain weight. For that "winning edge," coaches and athletes alike are learning that weight control, and the nutritional practices to achieve ideal weight, must be scientifically managed, just like every other aspect of athletic preparation.

Weight control and energy management practices should be of concern to all coaches, not just coaches in sports which have weight categories or sports which require tremendous amounts of energy. When athletes are at their ideal weight and are properly fueled, their performance is inevitably better—regardless of the sport being played.

Earl Edwards and Ken Willard, both professional football players, learned the value of scientifically managed weight control programs. Using body composition procedures developed by sport physiologists, the proportion of muscle and fat on Earl and Ken was computed. Earl, a defensive lineman, was 20% fat, and Ken, a running back, was 18% fat. When they learned that a running back's ideal fat weight is 6-8% and a defensive lineman's is 13-15%, they both went on diets. Earl dropped to 16% and Ken reduced to 11.5%.

According to their coaches, these men played better than ever after

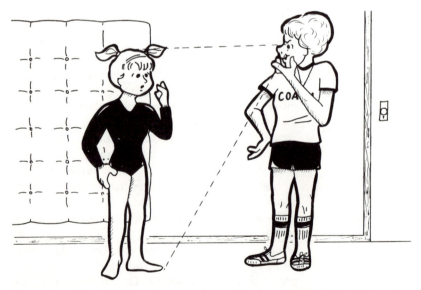

Figure 1.1. *The old binocular scanning method or "eyeball" technique is a poor way to determine the athlete's ideal weight.*

losing the weight. Ken was particularly elated, claiming that not since junior high school had he been able to execute some of the moves he now could do.

Peg Neppel, a long distance runner, also knows the value of managing an athlete's weight. In her freshman year at Iowa State University, her running times were poor—even slower than when she was in high school. At first, Peg didn't know what was wrong, but she eventually realized that the weight she had gained since high school was unneeded fat. She stepped up her training and cut out the desserts. As her percent fat decreased, her times improved and improved, so much that Peg Neppel set the 10,000 meter record for American women.

Gymnast Nadia Comaneci has also experienced the impact of weight control on her career. In the 1976 Olympics, her optimal body efficiency was reflected in phenomenal performances, but in the months after the Olympics, she grew taller and put on weight. As a result, her performances suffered and only after a lot of hard work on technique and weight control was Nadia able to regain championship form for the 1980 Olympics.

Earl Edwards, Ken Willard, Peg Neppel, and Nadia Comaneci are only a few of the many athletes who have discovered the importance of proper weight control, but countless other athletes, and their coaches, have not. Of all sports, wrestling has the most notorious reputation for poor weight control and energy management practices. Although the abuse is sometimes exaggerated, the bad "rap" is not without foundation, as Davey Samuelson's story illustrates.

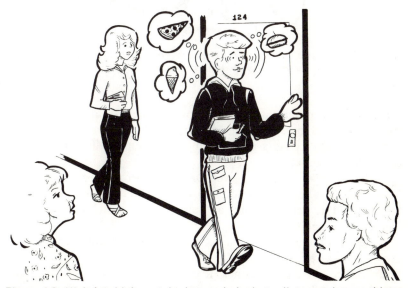

Figure 1.2. *High fat, high protein, low carbohydrate diets can leave athletes weak, dazed, and unable to concentrate.*

When Davey was faced with the task of losing 19 lbs—from 145 to 126—in 6 days to "make weight" for his Friday wrestling match, he decided to try a new high fat, high protein, low carbohydrate diet about which he had read. After 3 days of nothing but chicken legs, Davey found himself walking around in a daze, bumping into doors and walls, and daydreaming in school. Practices were a disaster! Without his usual energy, he was "hammered" by teammates who seldom could beat him, which then put the coach on his back.

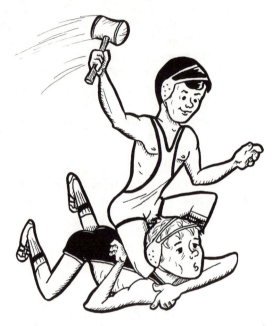

Figure 1.3. *Wrestlers who use rapid weight loss techniques frequently find themselves being "hammered" in the waning minutes of practice or a match.*

Although the diet was working, on Wednesday afternoon Davey still had 7 lbs to lose. So he decided to stop drinking water. By Thursday, he couldn't pass a water fountain without hallucinations of a giant glass of milk.

Friday morning, a sunken-eyed Davey popped a "pee green" pill to help squeeze out even more water. Irritable and depressed, Davey was having trouble getting along at home and school. He mostly just wanted to be left alone.

Weigh-in time arrived Friday at 5 p.m. Davey had been in a sauna most of the afternoon, and as he stripped off his clothes to weigh, his body looked like a pink prune. He delicately stepped on the scale, exhaled completely in hopes of shedding air weight, and prayed fervently as the scale's balance bar hovered near the top. The referee bent for-

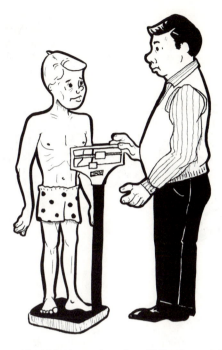

Figure 1.4. *Davey need not look so glum, he will "make weight"—this time. But will his shriveled body be able to wrestle?*

ward for a closer look, then smiled. With the clearance of a gnat's eyelash, Davey had made weight for another week.

He leapt from the scale, charged to his locker, and gulped a half gallon of gatorade, devoured two oranges, and inhaled four chocolate bars. Soon he would be ready to wrestle. . . or so he thought!

Davey's body was far from being ideally prepared to wrestle, but many wrestlers follow this or similar weight loss procedures week after week. In chapters 5 and 6, we will explain why high fat, high protein, low carbohydrate diets in combination with dehydration are doubly dangerous and deprive athletes of their peak performance potential.

Stephanie Smith, a member of her collegiate volleyball team, also wanted to lose weight. Her weight problem stemmed from her academic problems. The more she worried about staying eligible, the more she ate. As the pounds went on, the poorer she played volleyball, which she now worried about too. And the more she ate.

Finally, Stephanie's coach, who had noticed the weight gain, urged her to lose a few pounds. In desperation, she went on a 3-day fast and severely restricted her water intake. After three vigorous matches on Saturday afternoon, Stephanie found herself in the hospital. Intravenous fluids were necessary to restore the fluid and food balance she had disrupted with her crazy weight control scheme. In chapter 7, you

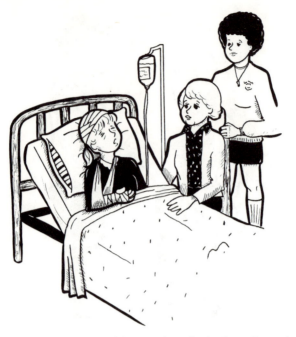

Figure 1.5. *Unfortunately some athletes unknowingly abuse the water and fuel needs of their bodies and require medical aid in restoring the appropriate balances.*

will learn how Stephanie should have properly lost the weight she had gained.

Not all athletes, of course, want to lose weight, as Larry Jansen can well tell you. After a discouraging football season in which he seldom played, Larry met with his coach to find out what he could do over the summer to better his chances of playing next season. He was just too small his coach explained.

Determined to play, Larry went to work on his problem. He ate everything in sight, taking special care to pack away lots of eggs, bacon, and red meat (which, he thought, builds muscle.) All summer long, he forced himself to eat gigantic milk shakes with bananas, eggs, nuts, and coconut. He fortified these concoctions with lecithin and other supplements such as wheat germ, zinc, vitamin E, and Brewer's yeast.

This delightful ordeal helped Larry gain 32 lbs. But when football season arrived, much to Larry's dismay, he did not pass the physical examination. His blood pressure was too high! Most of Larry's gain was fat weight and probably would not have helped him play better even if it had not sidelined him with high blood pressure. In chapter 8, we will explain how to properly gain muscle weight, *not* fat weight.

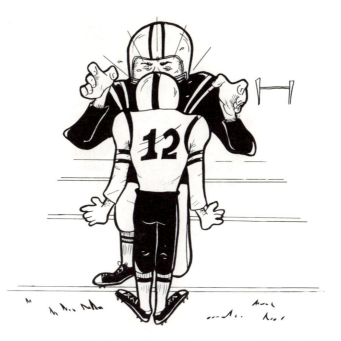

Figure 1.6. *Even if the opponents tower over your athletes, don't let your players succumb to the temptation of becoming human garbage disposals. Simply being bigger (fatter) will not help them play better!*

"Moose" McGraw was a litle smarter than Larry Jansen; he knew the difference between muscle and fat weight. After a sensational season this past year, and rumors surfacing that he would be a Heisman Trophy contender this coming season, Moose decided a little more muscle weight would help him be even better.

When the new season began though, he was hampered with a nagging toe injury. For several weeks, the medical staff thought it was turf toe, but finally discovered Moose had, of all things, gout. He had been consuming so much protein supplement that the uric acid produced by the metabolized protein rose to excessive levels in his body. His kidneys were unable to remove all the uric acid, so his body took it out on his toe.

Moose's bout with gout is an example of the "more is better" myth that traps athletes seeking to build their body with food supplements. In chapter 4, you will learn why athletes need not and should not consume excessive quantities of protein or vitamins.

A Coach's Responsibility

Most coaches acknowledge the importance of weight control and nutrition for good athletic performance, but many candidly admit that they really do little to directly assist their athletes. Why?

Perhaps coaches find it difficult to wade through the morass of nutritional and weight control literature which appears in newspapers, on television, and in countless magazine articles and books. Separating fact from fiction with all the fad diets and supposed magical potions is no easy task. Coaches also may be uncertain whether weight control methods intended for middle-aged adults are appropriate for energy-demanding athletes. Or perhaps coaches are more familiar with the traditions of their sport than with the research findings of sport scientists. For example, do you still follow such practices as:

- the supposed high-energy steak and egg meal the morning of the big game
- mandatory consumption of salt tablets on hot days
- candy bars and oranges for quick energy
- expensive liquid concoctions thought to be superior to water
- refraining from drinking cold water
- protein pills as dietary supplements

Are these the best practices? Can you tell fact from fiction in weight control and energy management techniques for your athletes?

Coach John Stringer can. Bill Ferguson weighed 150 lbs when he reported for wrestling after completing a successful football season. Coach Stringer computed Bill's percent body fat using procedures described in chapter 2: It was 14%. Knowing that the ideal percent fat is 5-7% for a champion wrestler, Coach Stringer explained to Bill that his *optimal* weight class would be the 137 lb category. Through a carefully planned weight control program supervised by Coach Stringer, Bill slowly lost the weight over a 3-month period.

Coach Stringer also urged Gary Landers, who had been wrestling at the 103 lb classification, to move up a weight class by gaining 7 lbs. Gary had only 3% body fat and was just too weak at the lower weight class. Gary followed the coach's advice, and even though he did not have a spectacular season in terms of winning, he enjoyed wrestling more than ever because he was not constantly starving.

The knowledge Coach Stringer has is found in the remaining chapters of this book. We will show you how to determine the ideal weight for each of your athletes and will give you the essential information you need to help your athletes adjust their weight safely and properly in order to achieve the right proportion of bone, muscle, and fat. We will explain how to meet the nutritional needs, not of sedentary middle-aged adults, but of high energy-consuming athletes. And we will dispel many nutritional myths which abound in sport.

In subsequent chapters, you will learn about the vital role of water in athletic performance, when vitamins and mineral supplements are needed, and which foods are really high in energy. You also will learn about the effectiveness of the high-energy, superfuel carbohydrate diet. In short, we will present weight control and energy management practices which are not based on opinion or current nutritional fashion, but on scientifically proven facts.

Chapter 2
Appraising Ideal Weight

In the last chapter we discussed the importance of *ideal weight*. Now let's learn more about it and find out how to measure it.

Ideal weight is highly individualized. It is the weight which allows an athlete to function optimally in his or her chosen sport. **There is no one ideal body weight for all athletes.** What is an ideal weight for one athlete may be completely inappropriate for another.

Helping athletes achieve their ideal weight is more complicated than simply manipulating how much they weigh when they get on the scale. For example, gymnasts should not only minimize body weight, but should also maximize their strength to enhance their skill and prevent injuries. Similarly, wrestlers should compete at the weight class in which their strength, endurance, and skill are optimal. Achievement of these objectives depends upon understanding of three basic facts.

FACT 1: The body's weight is composed of many different constituents. Muscle tissue, nerve tissue, bone, ligaments, tendons, skin, minerals, and fat are all part of the body's composition. For convenience, authorities have consolidated these

11

constituents into two major component parts: fat tissue and lean or muscle tissue. This means that body weight is composed of lean body weight (sometimes called fat free weight) and fat weight. Thus:

Body Weight = Lean Body Weight + Fat Weight

FACT 2: Not all of the body's constituents contribute equally to the body's weight. For example, all of the constituents of lean body weight are more dense than the fat tissue. Density refers to the mass of a substance relative to its volume. To illustrate this idea, imagine a balance scale with a 1-lb lead pellet on one of the balance trays. The container with the 1-lb lead pellet would not need to be very large. Now imagine you balanced the lead pellet with a pound of feathers, as shown in Figure 2.1; it would take a very large container to hold them. The reason for this disparity in the size of the containers is due to the difference in the density of lead and feathers. Lead is quite dense; it has a relatively small volume relative to its mass (weight). Feathers, on the other hand, are not dense; they have a large volume relative to their mass.

The body's lean body weight and fat weight also vary in density. Lean tissue is more dense than fat tissue. Consequently, it is possible to have two individuals with the same height and weight, but with completely different body dimensions, such as the two girls in Figure 2.2. The girl on the right has 30% fat and obviously larger dimensions than the girl on the left, who is only 20% fat.

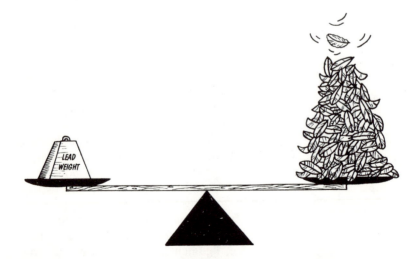

Figure 2.1. *Lead is more dense than feathers, so a pound of feathers will take up more space than a pound of lead.*

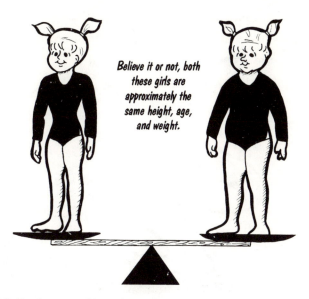

Believe it or not, both these girls are approximately the same height, age, and weight.

Figure 2.2. *Fat tissue and lean tissues vary in density, and so simply looking at scale weight can be misleading.*

Because of this difference in the contribution of fat tissue and lean tissue to the body's weight, more is required than simply monitoring the scales to help athletes achieve their ideal weight. The coach and athlete need to be aware of whether fat weight or lean weight is being lost or gained.

FACT 3: Not all of the body's constituents contribute equally to sport performance potential. The contraction of the various muscles used to propel the body and implements such as rackets and balls depends upon the muscles receiving guiding signals from the nervous system. The nervous system also regulates the work of the heart to pump blood to the muscles which also is fundamental to the execution of sport activities. Without strong bones, the contractile forces of the skeletal muscles could not be used for throwing, running, and jumping. Because the nerves, skeletal muscles, heart, blood vessels, and bones are all part of the lean body weight, it is readily apparent that the lean tissues are essential to the performance of physical activities. On the other hand, a large quantity of body fat does not help performance. For example, in a study of 835 high school wrestlers by Tcheng and Tipton,[1] the average body fat was 8%, but the 224 state finalists had body fat contents ranging between 4 to 6%. Obviously, the better or more successful wrestlers were also the leaner wrestlers.

---

[1]Tcheng, T., & Tipton, C. Iowa wrestling study: Anthropometric measurements and the prediction of a ''minimal'' body weight for high school wrestlers. *Medicine and Science in Sports*, 1973, **5**(1), 1-10.

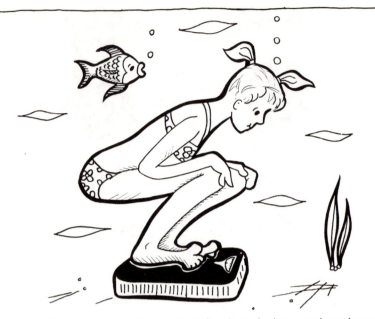

Figure 2.3. *Underwater weighing is more than just placing a scale underwater; it is a scientific way of using land weight and underwater weight to calculate body density.*

Body Composition Appraisal

To implement a scientifically managed weight control program, you need some means for determining the athlete's body composition. In other words, you need to find out what percentage of the athlete's body weight is fat weight and what percentage is lean tissue. Such information will allow you to know if the athlete has excess fat weight or if additional lean weight needs to be gained.

Well and good, you say, but how practical is it to appraise body composition? Although a number of things need to be considered and a margin of error exists, you can quite readily learn to compute your athletes' fat weight and lean body weight. These considerations and the procedures for appraising body composition are presented next.

Hydrostatic Weighing

The most accurate technique for appraising body composition is called hydrostatic or underwater weighing. With this procedure, the athletes are submerged in water to obtain their "underwater" weight. Once the underwater weight is obtained along with the land weight, a series of calculations are computed to determine body density.

Although submerging athletes in water may seem like a strange practice, underwater weight permits the calculation of body density because fat is less dense than lean tissue. Consequently, athletes with a high percent of fat will weigh less underwater than athletes with the same body weight but a lower percent of fat. For the same reason, people with a lot of fat float more easily than lean people. The fat is buoyant in water because it is less dense than the water.

Despite its accuracy, underwater weighing is not widely used because the equipment is costly, experienced technicians are needed, and a considerable amount of time is required. Scientists, therefore, have developed more practical techniques for use by physicians and coaches. One technique measures the skinfold at certain points on the body and the other takes anthropometrical measurements on the body.

The Skinfold Method

Skinfold procedures, or "pinch tests" (see Figure 2.4) as they are sometimes called, entail measuring the distance across a fold of skin as shown in Figure 2.5. In pinching a "fold" of skin, you also pick up the subcutaneous (meaning "beneath the skin") fat. Scientists have learned that about 50% of the body's fat is stored just beneath the skin. This knowledge is used to predict the body's total fat composition.

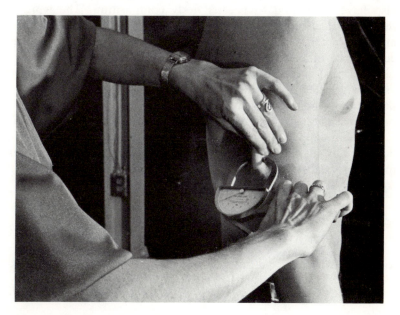

Figure 2.4. *The triceps skinfold.*

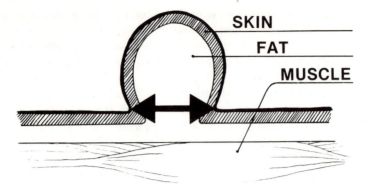

Figure 2.5. *The skinfold caliper is used to measure the thickness of the subcutaneous fat in a "pinch" of skin.*

Although the skinfold method is a relatively simple idea, its application requires skill and knowledge. One of the major difficulties with the method is that a number of factors seem to influence where people deposit subcutaneous fat. Children deposit fat in different places than adults, males deposit fat in different sites than females, and nonathletes deposit fat differently than athletes. Recent research even shows that different types of athletes deposit fat differently. Such variability means that different skinfold sites must be used according to the age, sex, and sport of the specific athlete.

In addition to skinfold procedures, anthropometrical measurements also have been used to predict body composition. The word anthropometrical refers to the measurement of human beings, and so anthropometrical techniques include measurements of the circumference of limbs or the trunk (for example, abdominal girths, biceps girths) and measurements of skeletal diameters (for example, ankle width and knee width). The use of such measurements in the prediction of body composition capitalizes on the known relationship between skeletal size and the total amount of lean tissue in the body.

The skin caliper method of appraising body composition is fully described in this chapter. It is the more general and hence more useful method for most sports. We will present specific procedures for the following athletic groups using the caliper method:

Females	**Males**
9-12 years old	9-12 years old
13-16 years old	13-16 years old
17 and up (see chapter 11)	17 and up (see chapter 11)

There are better body composition appraisal methods for certain sports groups. The anthropometrical method is best for college-aged women gymnasts and a variant of the caliper method is better for college-aged football players. These two methods are described in Appendix A and B. For all other sports, the caliper method is the best practical procedure available today.

Skinfold Measurement

Preliminaries

Although the skinfold method is proven to be valid, it is not fail-safe. The skill of the person taking the measurements greatly determines its validity. Using skin calipers is a motor skill just like shooting freethrows or driving tee shots in golf. An uncoached beginner will be less accurate than a well-coached, experienced veteran. So, we will coach you in the proper use of the calipers and then urge you to practice taking many measurements.

The first thing you need to do, obviously, is acquire a skin caliper. We have listed the sources for purchasing calipers in Appendix C with their approximate cost. The quality of the caliper you purchase is also important. If less expensive calipers are used, the accuracy and consistency will suffer somewhat. However, a little practice can help improve this accuracy, and instructions for using one such caliper are presented in Appendix J.

We also must point out that the equations used to compute body composition are based on averages compiled from many individuals. It is possible, therefore, that a given athlete's body build might be such that the equation is not entirely accurate for him or her. Even under the best of circumstances, there is as much as a 3% error in the predictive equations we present. We mention this margin of error only to emphasize that common sense and good judgment must accompany your use of the caliper and calculator, not to discourage your use of this method. Indeed, we strongly urge that you employ them to replace the less accurate eyeball method.

Caliper Method

Many different methods have been developed for using skin calipers. The specific procedure described here is well documented and relatively simple. It requires you to take two skinfold measurements: one from the triceps and one from the subscapula.

Both of these measurements are to be taken on the *right side* of the

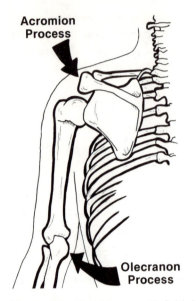

Acromion Process

Olecranon Process

Figure 2.6. The triceps skinfold is taken at the midpoint between the acromion process and the olecranon process.

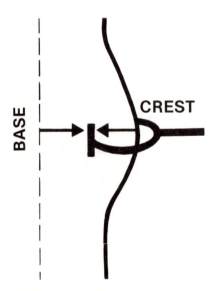

BASE

CREST

Figure 2.7. Position the caliper at the point of the fold where a true double thickness of skinfold fat exists, which will be approximately midway between the crest and base of the skinfold.

body on all athletes. You must take considerable care in locating the precise site for the measurement because the accuracy of the test depends on it. For the triceps measurement, locate the point over the triceps muscle that is exactly halfway between the elbow (olecranon process) and the shoulder (acromion process of the scapula). (See Figure 2.6 for the location of these structures.)

You may wish to use a tape measure to help locate the halfway point. Once you have located this point, firmly grasp the skin between the left (right, if you're left-handed) thumb and forefinger and lift up the skin with its underlying fat tissue (see Figure 2.4). The skinfold should be parallel to the longitudinal axis of the arm. Be careful that you do not have muscle tissue in your skinfold. To prevent this from occurring, have the athlete make a fist. When the triceps muscle is contracted, you should not be able to feel any muscle tissue in the skinfold.

Once you are sure that you have the right site and that you don't have any muscle tissue, have the athlete relax the arm; then take the caliper in your right hand and open its "jaws." Place the contact surfaces 1 centimeter (cm) below the fingers of your left hand (right, if left-handed). The idea is to position the caliper at the point of the fold where a true double thickness of skinfold fat exists (which will be approximately midway between the crest and base of the skinfold, as shown in Figure 2.7).

Now slowly release the lever on the caliper so that the "jaws" are able to exert their full tension on the skinfold. The needle on the caliper dial will drop slightly. When the needle stops moving (1-2 seconds after releasing your grip), read the dial to the nearest 0.5 millimeter (mm). Record this value on the score sheet, which is shown in Table 2.1. Repeat this procedure two more times on the same site so that you can record three consecutive readings.

The second skinfold to be taken is the subscapular skinfold. You can find the site for this skinfold by locating the fold of skin which is 1 cm below the inferior angle of the right scapula (the bottom of the right "shoulder blade" as shown in Figure 2.8). The exact angle of the skin-

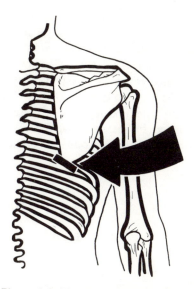

Figure 2.8. *The subscapular skinfold is taken over the inferior angle of the right scapula (the bottom of the right "shoulder blade").*

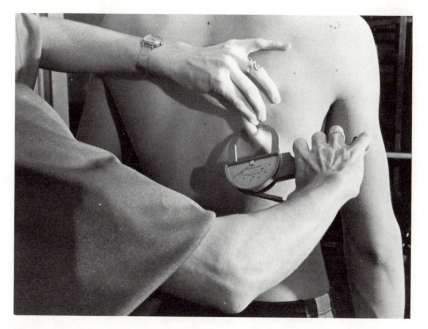

Figure 2.9. *The subscapular skinfold.*

fold depends somewhat on the individual, so locate the natural fold of the skin (see Table 2.2). Once you have located the skinfold site, use the caliper to take the actual measurement in exactly the same way that you did for the triceps measurement (see Figure 2.7).

Once you have finished using the caliper, the most difficult part of measuring body composition is behind you. All that remains to be done is to predict your athlete's ideal weight, which can be accomplished by performing the following five steps. The Ideal Weight Recording Form found in Table 2.1 will make it easy.

Table 2.1

Ideal Weight Recording Form

Name _____ Age _____

Date _____ Weight _____ lbs

Ideal Weight Prediction _____ lbs   Weight to Lose/Gain _____ lbs

Skinfolds

	#1	#2	#3	Average
Triceps	_____ mm	_____ mm	_____ mm	_____ mm
Subscapular	_____ mm	_____ mm	_____ mm	_____ mm

Predicted % fat as read from the appropriate skinfold table = _____ %

Body Wt. × Fat = Fat Weight   Body Weight − Fat Weight = LBW

_____ × _____ = _____   _____ − _____ = _____

$$\text{Ideal Body Weight} = \frac{\text{LBW}}{(100\% - \text{Ideal \% Fat})}$$

$$\frac{}{(100\% -)} = \underline{} \text{lbs}$$

$$\frac{}{} = \underline{} \text{lbs}$$

Step 1

Determine the average skinfold value for both the triceps and subscapular measurement. Simply add the three triceps measurements and divide by 3.

Step 2

Select the appropriate skinfold table (see Table 2.2) on the basis of the age and sex of the athlete.

Step 3

Find the average triceps skinfold value on the "triceps line" of Table 2.2 and the average subscapular skinfold on the "subscapula line." Use a straight edge or ruler to then connect the two skinfold values. The point at which the ruler intersects the "% fat line" on the table gives the predicted percent fat value. Record this number in the appropriate place on the recording form.

Step 4

Determine the athlete's lean body weight. Because body weight is comprised of fat weight plus lean body weight, the lean body weight may be determined by subtracting the fat weight from the body weight. The formula presented in Table 2.1 should help you with these calculations. For example, let's say that Eric, a cross country runner, has a percent fat of 14% and a body weight of 120 lbs.

$$\text{Body Weight} \times \text{\% Fat} = \text{Fat Weight}$$

$$120 \text{ lbs} \times .14 = 14.8 \text{ lbs}$$

When we do the rest of the computations, we find that Eric's lean body weight is 105.2 lbs.

$$\text{Body Weight} - \text{Fat Weight} = \text{Lean Body Weight}$$

$$120 \text{ lbs} - 14.8 \text{ lbs} = 105.2 \text{ lbs}$$

Step 5

Now we are ready to determine the athlete's ideal body weight. The formula for doing so is:

Ideal Body Weight = Lean Body Weight ÷ (100% − Ideal % Fat)

This formula introduces a new term, *ideal percent fat.*Remember, we

Table 2.2

Skinfold Tables For Children

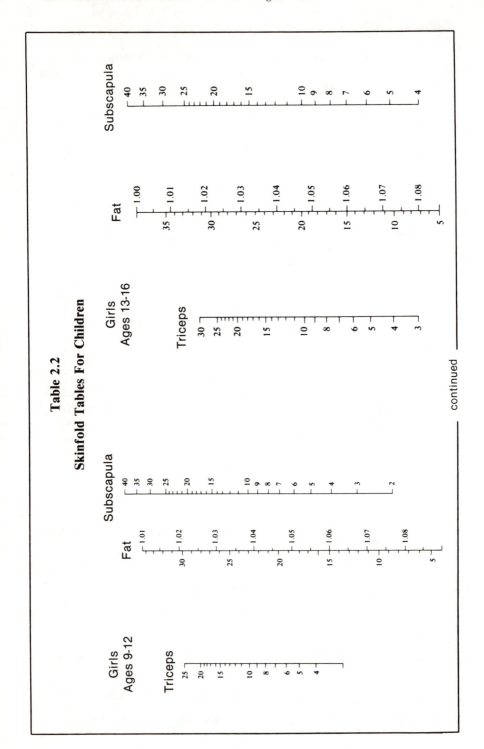

continued

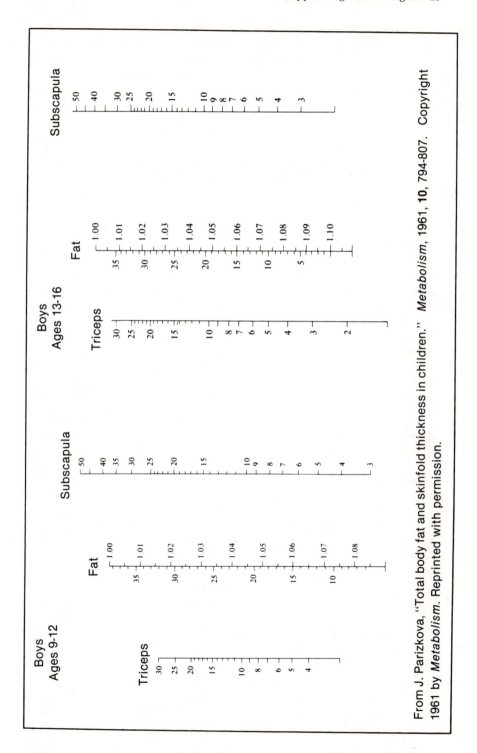

From J. Parizkova, "Total body fat and skinfold thickness in children." *Metabolism*, 1961, **10**, 794-807. Copyright 1961 by *Metabolism*. Reprinted with permission.

said that ideal weight is an individual matter, depending upon both the athlete and the sport. Although we obviously cannot tell you the ideal weight for a particular athlete, we can tell you the typical ideal percent fat values for certain sports. These values are presented in Table 2.3. If your sport is not listed, select the sport that comes nearest to your type of activity.

Table 2.3

**Ideal Percent Fat Values for Young Athletes
in Various Sports and Activities**

| Sport | Ideal % Fat Values | |
	Male	Female
Baseball and softball	8-10%	10-12%
Basketball	7- 9%	7-11%
Distance running	5- 7%	5- 9%
Sprinters	6-10%	7-11%
Field events	10-14%	10-16%
Football		
Def. back	6- 8%	8-10%
Off. back	6- 8%	8-10%
Linebacker	13-15%	15-20%
Off. lineman and tight ends	13-15%	15-20%
Def. lineman	13-15%	15-20%
Gymnasts	5- 7%	5-10%
Soccer and field hockey	7- 9%	7-11%
Swimming	6-10%	6-12%
Volleyball	7- 9%	7-11%
Wrestling	5- 7%	7- 9%

From J.M. Kelly and J.D. Wickkister, "Ideal and actual percent fat by position." *The Physician and Sportsmedicine*, 1975, **3**(12), 38-42. Copyright 1975 by McGraw-Hill. Reprinted with permission.

Now let's do an example under the assumption that you are a cross-country coach. First, look up the ideal percent fat (5-7%) for distance runners in Table 2.3. We suggest that you use the higher of the two numbers when first computing ideal weight if the athlete is likely to need to lose weight and to use the lower number if the athlete is likely to need to gain weight. This makes it easier to reach the first goal. Then you should evaluate the weight loss or gain on an individual basis and later use the lower or upper value if it appears appropriate.

Thus, to complete the ideal body weight calculations for Eric, whose lean body weight, remember, is 105.2 lbs, subtract 7% from 100%.

$$1.00 - .07 = .93$$

This .93 is inserted into the denominator of the equation.

Ideal Body Weight = Lean Body Weight ÷ (100% − Ideal % Fat)

Ideal Body Weight = 105.2 lbs ÷ .93

Ideal Body Weight = 113.1 lbs

Because Eric's weight is 120 lbs, he needs to lose 7 lbs of fat, reducing his body weight to 113 lbs for optimal efficiency in cross country running.

Table 2.4

Completed Ideal Weight Recording Form

Name ___*Rita Caller*___ Age ___*14 yrs.*___

Date ___*Sept. 1980*___ Weight _____ Height _____inches

Sport ___*Gymnastics*___ Ideal % Fat ___*5-7%*___

Ideal Weight Prediction ___*113*___lbs   Weight to Lose/Gain ___*12*___lbs

Skinfolds	#1	#2	#3	Average
Triceps	*6.5* mm	*6* mm	*5.5* mm	*6.0* mm
Subscapular	*8.0* mm	*8.0* mm	*8.0* mm	*8.0* mm

Predicted % fat as read from the appropriate skinfold table = ___*15.5*___ %

Body Wt. × Fat = Fat Weight   Body Weight − Fat Weight = LBW

___*125 lbs*___ × ___*.155*___ = *19.37 lbs*   ___*125 lbs*___ − ___*19.37 lbs*___ = ___*105.6 lbs*___

$$\text{Ideal Body Weight} = \frac{\text{LBW}}{(100\% - \text{Ideal \% Fat})}$$

$$\text{Ideal Body Weight (lbs)} = \frac{}{(100\% - .07)}$$

$$\underline{\quad 113 \quad}\text{lbs} = \frac{105.6\ lbs}{.93}$$

Let's do one more example, but this time we will do all of the calculations on the recording form in Table 2.4. As you can see, our young gymnast Rita, has a predicted ideal weight of 113 lbs, which means that she must lose 12 lbs of fat weight.

Summary

You have now learned how to measure and compute body composition and how to calculate ideal weight. But knowing what your athletes' ideal weight should be is a long way from getting your athletes to reach that weight. First, you must help them to understand the importance of achieving their ideal weight. Then, you need to help educate your athletes to eat and drink properly in order to achieve their ideal weight safely and to maintain high energy levels. In the next four chapters, we will help you understand how athletes can achieve these goals. One simple way to do this is to share this book with them.

Chapter 3
Proteins, Vitamins, and Minerals

Advertisements in many sport magazines would have us believe that athletes benefit from the use of protein, vitamin, and mineral supplements— and that the more they take the better. In this chapter, we will explain what proteins, vitamins, and minerals are and what they do. And we will discuss how much of these substances athletes really need.

What are Proteins?

Proteins, which contain 20 or so amino acids, form the "building blocks" of life. The body uses these amino acids to form the framework of the various cells of our bodies. Amino acids are also the major component of enzymes (the chemicals which regulate life processes). Protein, therefore, is an important substance in our diet, but there is a limit to how much protein the body can safely use. No more than 10-20% of the calories we eat should come from protein. For the nonathlete, this means about 1-1.5 grams of protein per kilogram of weight. Because athletes burn more calories and are building and repairing more tissues than nonathletes, they should eat 1.5-2.0 grams of protein per kilogram of weight. This means that a 150-lb (70 kg) athlete should eat 1 cup of cottage cheese, a chicken breast, and a couple of glasses of milk to meet his protein needs. Most Americans already eat far more protein than this.

Many athletes and coaches believe that athletes need to consume more protein than the average person in order to build strong bones and muscles. This is a myth you need to dispel among your athletes. Convey to them that 1.5-2.0 grams of protein per kilogram of body weight is optimal; help them analyze foods like those shown in Appendix D to understand what 1.5-2.0 grams of proteins per kilogram of body weight means to them. For example, if Susan weighs 40 kg or 88 lbs (to convert pounds to kilograms, divide by 2.2), her protein requirement is between 60 grams (1.5g/kg × 40 kg = 60 g) and 80 grams per day. By looking at the protein content of the foods in Appendix D, you can show Susan that by drinking three glasses of milk and having a tuna fish sandwich, a couple of pieces of chicken, and yogurt snack, she can easily meet her protein requirement.

Your efforts to educate your athletes in this way begins their "nutritional conditioning"—a part of their training which is just as important as their "physical conditioning." This education will not only help your athletes play better, it's likely to help them develop eating habits which will let them live longer and happier. The "fat American" is not the result of an accident, the product of some

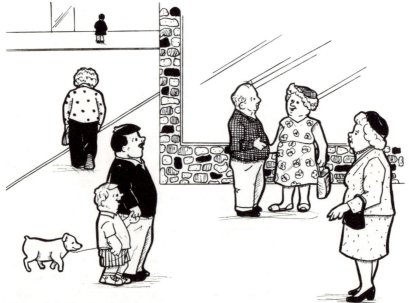

Figure 3.1. *The Fat American.*

foreign virus, nor the result of some genetic abnormality. Rather, obesity is a reflection of poor eating habits and lack of physical activity. Therefore, because sport places a premium on physical efficiency and energy management, you are in an ideal position as a coach to foster positive weight control and motivation habits.

What Happens When Too Much Protein is Eaten?

Unfortunately, many athletes are unaware of the dangers of eating too much protein. One of the problems with excessive protein consumption is that animal protein sources like red meat, whole milk, eggs, and most cheeses also contain large quantities of saturated fat. This "hidden fat" can contribute large numbers of unwanted calories. Furthermore, high levels of dietary saturated fat have been shown to be related to increased levels of blood fats and cholesterol as well as increased body fat, blood pressure, and coronary heart disease. Eating large quantities of fat is particularly dangerous if the athlete's family already has the tendency to have high blood pressure or a history of coronary heart disease. The high blood pressure problem is further aggravated by the large amount of salt often eaten with animal proteins. So athletes who eat large quantities of animal protein are not only likely to gain fat weight, they are also forming poor lifetime eating habits.

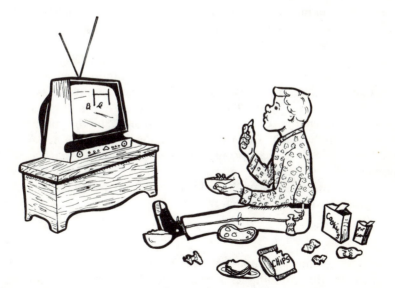

Figure 3.2. *Conditioning involves changing poor eating habits as well as physically training the body.*

Another fact which many young athletes don't know is that only so many amino acids can be used to make muscle tissue. Extra protein is *not* used for energy, but instead is converted into fat by the liver and is stored. Because fat is excess baggage and does not contribute to strength, power, or quickness, eating excessive amounts of protein only hinders athletic performance.

And don't forget "Moose" McGraw, who had his bout with gout from eating too much protein. When the liver converts excess protein to fat, the nitrogen part of the amino acid must be removed from the body. To do so, the liver makes uric acid out of this nitrogen substance so the kidney can excrete the uric acid in the urine. If the uric acid levels in the blood get too high while the kidney is trying to excrete the uric acid, gout may develop.

Another hidden problem associated with protein metabolism is dehydration or the loss of body water. This occurs because the kidneys must use water to form the urine in order to wash out the excess uric acid. This also explains *part* of why crash diets can result in rapid weight loss. During the crash dieting, the body's proteins are used for fuel, therefore producing uric acid. So water weight is lost as the kidneys remove uric acid from the blood.

What are Vitamins?

The word vitamin means vital. Vitamins are organic substances that are essential in minute quantities for specific chemical reactions in the cells. Because cells cannot manufacture these substances, they must be included in the food we eat.

Although many of the vitamins act as co-enzymes for the energy-releasing chemical reactions of the body, the vitamins themselves are not a direct source of energy. Thus, taking more vitamins does not ensure that the athlete will have more energy. The vitamins simply "spark" the energy-releasing processes involved in the burning of fuels within the cells. But this close relationship with the energy-producing reactions has prompted many to assume that vitamin supplements will enhance performance—the "more is better syndrome" again! So you can help educate your athletes about vitamins, let's look at what the research tells us.

Vitamin E

At various times, proponents of Vitamin E supplements have claimed that this vitamin increases stamina, improves circulation and the delivery of oxygen to the muscles, lowers cholesterol, prevents graying of hair, and cures infertility. Most of these claims are based upon animal research findings. For example, some years ago, a group of researchers devised a Vitamin E deficient diet, which they fed to rats. Among the symptoms the rats exhibited was sterility. When Vitamin E was returned to their diet, they became potent again.

The temptation to generalize these findings to say that Vitamin E cures infertility in humans is great, but follow-up studies with humans have revealed that the millions of people, especially athletes who spend enormous sums of money on Vitamin E capsules, solutions, fortifiers, skin lotions, and other products are doing so needlessly. Scientists have failed to verify that large Vitamin E supplements are in any way related to better athletic performance. Although it is true that athletes may require more Vitamin E than nonathletes, (see Table 3.1 for recommended vitamin dosages), remember that athletes also eat more than nonathletes. Thus, by eating nutritious foods, an optimal amount of Vitamin E can be consumed. Let your athletes know that vegetable oils, unrefined cereal products (especially wheat germ), and eggs are good sources of Vitamin E. White bread, junk food, and soda pop contain relatively little Vitamin E, which robs athletes' bodies of endurance and muscle tone. Incidentally, Vitamin E helps protect the lungs from the effects of pollution.

Can an athlete get too much Vitamin E? At one time it was thought that Vitamin E was nontoxic, but recent findings indicate that overzealous supplementation (above 2000 I.U./kg) may be harmful. Encourage athletes to eat proper diets high in Vitamin E, preventing the need for supplements.

Table 3.1

Recommended Vitamin Dosages For Various Athletes

Vitamin (mg/day)	Nonathletes	Power and Strength Athletes	Endurance Athletes
A	1.5	2	2
B_1	1.5	4-6	6-10
B_2	2	3	4
C	75	100-200	100-300
D	2	2	2
E	5	7	10

From J. Nocker and H. Glatzel, *Die Ernahrung Des Sportlers*. West Germany: Nationales Olympisches Komitee für Deutschland, 1963. Copyright 1963 by the Nationales Olympisches Komitee für Deutschland.

The Vitamin B Complex

Although a number of vitamins constitute the Vitamin B complex, only vitamins B_1, B_2, Niacin, and B_{12}, seem to be required in greater than normal quantities for athletes. The exact requirements are determined by the nature and intensity of the training regime and competitive schedule (see Table 3.1).

The athlete's requirement for Vitamin B_1 or thiamine is higher than that of nonathletes because this vitamin plays a very important role in the glucose-"burning" chemical reactions. Therefore, the more calories burned, as in training, the greater the body's need for thiamine. Vitamin B_2 (lactoflavin or riboflavin) also plays an important function in the energy-metabolism or energy-releasing processes. In addition to its role in carbohydrate metabolism, niacin, still another of the B vitamins, is indispensible for fat and protein metabolism. Consequently, the dietary requirements for these B complex vitamins do increase with training, but usually this increased need is met by increased caloric consumption. If, however, the athlete is on a restricted caloric intake, supplementation may be necessary. In this case, a good multiple vitamin is the best approach, because it contains all the vitamins in a "balanced" fashion.

Vitamin B_{12} has an antianemic effect; in addition, it has some special effects on the metabolism of amino acids (the component parts of proteins) and the nervous system. Again, higher than normal doses are recommended, particularly for athletes performing at high altitudes. These increased B_{12} needs should be met, however, through eating more foods high in B_{12} rather than taking supplements. Athletes on reducing diets may wish to take a multiple vitamin.

An interesting paradox exists for many teenage athletes. Typically, young athletes are aware that carbohydrates are a rapid source of energy because they have frequently heard that "sugar is quick energy." So, they happily stuff themselves with sugar-laden junk foods under the pretense that they are consuming quick energy. What these athletes fail to realize is that the carbohydrate, or in other words, the sugar in the junk foods, actually destroys Vitamin B in the intestine. This is because Vitamin B is required to carry the sugar from the intestine into the blood.

Consumption of most sources of complex sugars or carbohydrates, such as cereals and vegetables does not present this problem because those foods contain more Vitamin B than it takes to digest them. This is not the case, however, with junk foods. Consequently, athletes who fulfill their energy needs with junk foods run the risk of vitamin deficiency. In fact, this situation is becoming alarmingly common among teenagers in general. No athlete can hope to achieve his or her optimal performance capabilities under such conditions. Thus, you can help

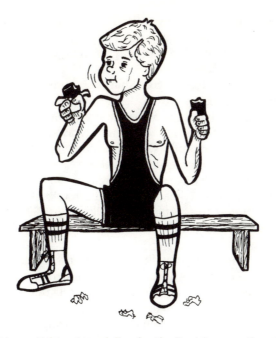

Figure 3.3. *Many athletes have fallen for the "quick energy" myth.*

athletes by providing them with a well thought-out nutritional conditioning program. A balanced diet is a much better approach to nutrition than encouraging youngsters to "pop vitamin pills." Such a practice merely reinforces the belief that pills solve our problems.

Vitamin C

Vitamin C is another vitamin which has received considerable attention recently. Because it has been suggested that doses of 10 to 100 times the amounts available in the most nutritious diet will be effective in preventing or shortening the duration of the common cold, some people are taking large doses of Vitamin C. Such supplementation is still controversial because some studies have failed to show that Vitamin C has either effect in normal individuals.

Why should Vitamin C alleviate cold symptoms? Because in test tubes, Vitamin C detoxifies histamine, a product that is released in the body in response to various stresses (including the common cold). Although this occurs in the test tube, we are not sure of the extent to which it occurs in the living human. But because athletes constantly subject themselves to the stress of physical training, it has been theorized that Vitamin C supplementation can be valuable to them. Furthermore, ample evidence supports the important role of ascorbic acid or Vitamin C in collagen synthesis. Collagen is an important constituent of the connective tissues of the body. The athlete in training is in constant need of collagen synthesis to strengthen existing connective tissue and to develop new tissues.

In light of these biological contributions, Ludvig Prokop, an East German physician, has proposed that the Vitamin C requirement of athletes and hard laborers is substantially greater than that of the average person. He suggests that athletes involved in endurance training, such as wrestlers, gymnasts, and ice skaters, who are training and running to maintain body weight, should increase Vitamin C intake to between 2 to 2.85 mg per kg of body weight or .90 to 1.29 mg per lb of body weight. This would mean that for the 100-lb athlete, 90-129 mg of Vitamin C should be consumed each day; for the 154 lb athlete in training, however, this quantity should be increased to 138-178 mg per day.

Prokop has also stated that Vitamin C in its natural form, in fruit juices for instance, is clearly superior to synthetic ascorbic acid. He has hypothesized that this superiority is probably due to the fact that, in nature, the ascorbic acid is consumed in conjunction with other naturally occurring substances which have a stabilizing effect. Thus, once again, the preferred method for increasing vitamin consumption is to eat greater quantities of fruits, vegetables, and whole grains. For the athlete involved in weight reduction, multivitamin preparations are much better than taking high dosages of individual vitamins.

Vitamin A

This vitamin makes a number of contributions to body functions. It helps maintain the health of the cells in the membranes which line the nasal passages and bronchial tubes (to the lungs) so that these membranes can protect you against cold, flu, smoke, and smog. Vitamin A also helps the body cope with the stress of training. Because of these important functions, athletes require slightly more Vitamin A than nonathletes (see Table 3.1). To ensure that your athletes get enough of this vitamin, have them eat orange, yellow, and green fruits and vegetables such as carrots, sweet potatoes, spinach, apricots, and cantaloupe.

Vitamin A is a fat soluble vitamin, meaning that unused quantities are stored in the body's fat; therefore excessive doses of Vitamin A can be toxic. Vitamins B and C are water soluble, and thus, are washed out of the body in the urine. Although it's very difficult to overdose on carrots, more and more physicians are reporting overdoses from Vitamin A pills.

Should Athletes Take Vitamin Pills?

We have repeatedly emphasized that taking separate pills for each of the vitamins is not conducive to good nutritional conditioning. Optimal body function is not just dependent upon taking in vitamins, but these vitamins must be available in the right combinations and quantities. This is why we advocate eating rather than "pill popping" as the foundation for nutritional conditioning. Foods, with their naturally available vitamins and nutrients, are the best way of meeting the body's needs as well as assuring that vitamin overdoses do not occur.

The possible exception to this emphasis on food is the smaller, lighter athlete involved in weight reduction. Dietary vitamin supplements can be a real adjunct for these athletes who are watching their caloric consumption. In such cases, the "stress," multiple-vitamin preparations, with their emphasis on Vitamins C, B, and Fe, are most beneficial as long as you and the athlete's parents realize that a low body weight leaves the athlete more vulnerable to overdoses.

By now, you might be asking, "What's Fe?" It's iron, which is a mineral and our next topic.

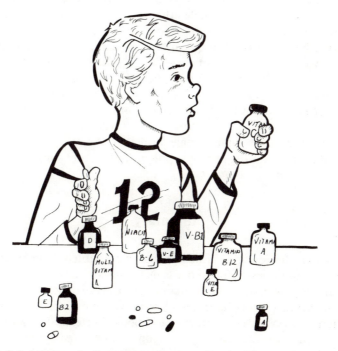

Figure 3.4. *Athletes don't need to rely upon vitamin pills.*

What are Minerals?

Minerals are the inorganic substances of the body. The body needs many minerals including sodium, potassium, chloride, calcium, phosphorus, magnesium, sulfur, and at least 14 trace minerals including iodine, flourine, and zinc. A detailed discussion of sodium, potassium, and chloride is presented in chapter 6. Calcium, phosphorous, and magnesium are necessary for the development of strong bones, and even though the athlete's training will stimulate bone development, the necessary minerals can be obtained through a normal balanced diet. For example, ample quantities of calcium may be obtained from milk and a variety of such plant foods as broccoli, spinach, and other leafy greens, whereas phosphorus and magnesium needs can be met by eating whole grain cereals, kidney beans, and lentils.

Our knowledge about the athlete's need for zinc and some of the other trace minerals is not yet complete. Zinc is required for growth, tissue repair, and blood cell formation—all functions of great importance to the athlete. To ensure ample zinc consumption, encourage your athletes to eat whole grains rather than purchase expensive zinc supplements.

To this point, we have not discussed any differences in dietary needs between young male and female athletes. This is because there simply are few differences. The young female athlete, however, because of her small size, does need to be careful in cutting calories so that protein and vitamin needs are not cut as well. Lighter male athletes should have this same concern, however. Female athletes who have begun menstruating may also need more iron than male athletes. Thus, the female athlete should be encouraged to maximize iron-rich foods in her diet (see Table 3.2). Furthermore, to prevent anemia, many physicians are suggesting that female athletes take supplemental iron. Remember, it's best if this iron is taken in the same supplement containing the Vitamins B and C.

Summary

Although the research indicates that most athletes can meet their protein, vitamin, and mineral needs by eating well-balanced meals, the vitamin supplement controversy continues to rage, particularly because recent reports have found some vitamin deficiencies among children in a variety of economic situations. For example, an investigation of the ascorbic acid consumption of the United States teenagers revealed that only 10.3% of the boys and 52.4% of the girls reached

Table 3.2

Typical Foods as Sources of Iron

Food	Size of Serving	Iron in Milligrams Per Average Serving	Iron in Milligrams Per 100 GM of Food
Liver			
Lamb, broiled	2 slices (75 gm)	13.4	17.9
Beef, fried	2 slices (75 gm)	6.6	8.8
Chicken, cooked	¼ c (50 gm)	4.3	8.8
Meats (lean or medium fat)			
Beef, round, cooked	1 large hamburger (85 gm)	3.0	3.5
Rib roast, cooked	3 slices (100 gm)	2.6	2.6
Pork, chop, cooked	1 medium large chop (80 gm)	2.5	3.1
Lamb, shoulder chop	1 chop, cooked (90 gm)	1.6	1.8
Baked beans, canned with			
pork and molasses	½ c (130 gm)	3.0	2.3
pork and tomato	½ c (130 gm)	2.3	1.8
Fruits, dried (uncooked)			
Apricots	4 halves (30 gm)	1.7	5.5
Prunes	4-5 medium (30 gm)	1.2	3.9
Figs	2 small (30 gm)	0.9	3.0
Raisins	2 tbsp (20 gm)	0.6	3.5
Legumes			
Soy beans, dry	½ c scant, cooked (30 gm dry)	2.5	8.4
Peanut butter	2 tbsp scant (30 gm)	0.6	2.0
Lima beans, fresh	½ c, cooked (80 gm)	2.0	2.5
Peas, fresh, green	½ c, cooked (80 gm)	1.4	1.8
Molasses, med.	1 tbsp (20 gm)	1.2	6.0
Eggs, whole	1 medium (50 gm)	1.2	2.3
Leafy vegetables			
Spinach	½ c, cooked (90 gm)	2.0	2.2
Beet greens	½ c, cooked (100 gm)	1.9	1.9
Chard	½ c, cooked (100 gm)	1.8	1.8
Kale, (leaves only)	½ c, cooked (55 gm)	0.9	1.6
Turnip greens	½ c, cooked (75 gm)	0.8	1.1
Vegetables			
Potatoes, sweet	1 medium baked (110 gm)	1.0	0.9
white	1 medium baked (100 gm)	0.7	0.7
Broccoli	⅔ c (100 gm)	0.8	0.8

continued

Table 3.2 (Cont.)

Typical Foods as Sources of Iron

| Food | Size of Serving | Iron in Milligrams | |
		Per Average Serving	Per 100 GM of Food
Brussel sprouts	5-6 medium (70 gm)	0.8	1.1
Cauliflower	¾ c, cooked (100 gm)	0.7	0.7
Carrots	⅔ c diced, cooked (100 gm)	0.6	0.6
String beans	¾ c cooked (100 gm)	0.6	0.6
Beets	2, 2-in diameter (100 gm)	0.5	0.5
Bread			
White, enriched	1 slice	0.6	2.5
Whole-wheat	1 slice	0.5	2.3
White, unenriched	1 slice	0.2	0.7
Cereals, whole grain (oats, corn, wheat, rice)	See label on package—range from 0.2 to 0.7 mg unenriched, up to 10 mg enriched, per serving		
Fresh fruits and fresh vegetables	100 gm serving, mostly	0.3-0.6	
Milk, whole, fluid, cow's,	½ pt or 8 oz (244 gm)	0.10	0.04
human	½ pt or 8 oz (244 gm)	0.24	0.1

Note. Most of these data are from *Composition of Foods*, Agriculture Handbook No. 8, US Department of Agriculture, 1963.

the standard recommendations of the Food and Nutrition Board. Such a dietary deficiency would certainly not be conducive to optimal athletic performance.

An examination of the reason or reasons for such low levels of dietary ascorbic acid indicates that the culprits are increased carbohydrate consumption (junk foods) as well as increased use of "practical" packaged foods. In other words, an ever-increasing percentage of our caloric consumption consists of "packaged" and "canned" foods which are high in calories and low in nutrient value. Furthermore, junk foods (candy bars, pop, cakes, and cookies) have become the major staple in the average American's diet. Consumption of these foods fills the individual's caloric needs but not the need for vitamins and minerals. If this situation exists for the average individual, for athletes with higher vitamin requirements, the possibility of vitamin inadequacies is indeed real.

Chapter 4
The Fuel Foods:
Carbohydrates and Fats

A well-balanced diet consists of a variety of constituents. We have already explained the role of proteins, vitamins, and minerals; now we will learn about the fuel foods: carbohydrates and fats.

Carbohydrates and fats are called "fuel foods" because they are taken into the cells of the body and burned to release energy. This combustion is possible because they consist of combinations of carbon, hydrogen, and oxygen molecules held together by bonds. When these bonds are broken by the chemical reactions which take place inside the cells, energy is released. This is similar to how gasoline burns.

During physical activity, the cells, particularly the muscle cells, must be capable of providing large quantities of energy. Obviously, then, coaches should have some understanding of how the fuel needs produced by physical activity are met. Thus, in this chapter we will focus on the relative contribution of fats and carbohydrates to the energy needs of athletes, as well as the physiological and psychological effects of inadequate fuel supplies.

Carbohydrates

Typically, athletes and coaches associate the word carbohydrate with "quick energy," but that's really a limited view of this important food category. For a better understanding of what carbohydrates can and cannot do for your athletes, let's take an in-depth look at this fuel food.

The word carbohydrate refers to the class of foods commonly known as sugars and starches. The basic structural unit of these fairly large molecules is a simple sugar or a short chain of carbon, hydrogen, and oxygen molecules. In other words, when we eat starchy food, such as bread or cereals, we are eating complex strings of simple sugars. Before the cells can use the energy in the starch, the string must be broken down to simple sugars. This is taken care of by the digestive system. Such simple sugars as glucose, fructose, and galactose then enter the blood stream from the intestine. Of these sugars, only glucose can be used directly by the cells. So as the blood passes through the liver, the liver ingeniously converts the other simple sugars to glucose.

Because cells can only "burn" glucose when it is inside them, the glucose must somehow enter the cells. A hormone called insulin plays an important role in this process. After carbohydrates are eaten and the glucose levels are elevated, the pancreas is "signaled" to release insulin. The insulin plays a role in carrying glucose into the muscle and other cells, except nerve cells. Glucose can enter nerve cells without insulin being present. As the glucose is taken into the cells, some is used and some is stored as a substance called glycogen. Just as there is a limit as to how much fuel you can put in your car's tank, there is also a limit as to how much glucose can be stored in the glycogen tanks. When the glycogen stores are filled, the remaining glucose that enters the cells is converted to fat, as shown in Figure 4.1.

Unfortunately, many athletes are unaware of this, so they overindulge in carbohydrate foods under the assumption that they are storing quick energy. The two main glycogen storage sites—the skeletal muscles and the liver—usually only store enough glucose to supply a sedentary individual's energy needs for about ½ day; trained athletes can store more. And if the procedures outlined in chapter 10 are followed, athletes can enlarge their glycogen storage capacity still further. But even these increased glycogen stores will only provide enough energy for 2-3 hours of intense exercise. So if you want your athletes to be capable of maximal effort for the entire game or throughout the entire tournament, some care must be taken to encourage the athlete to consume high carbohydrate foods, but not to exceed his or her caloric need (see chapter 7).

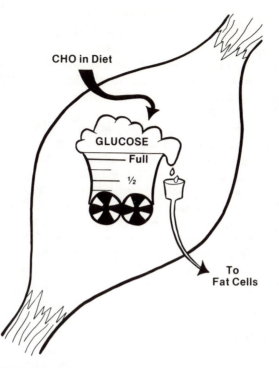

Figure 4.1. *Excess carbohydrates spill over into the fat storage tanks.*

Because extra carbohydrate Calories will be stored as fat, you must also pay attention to how long it takes to fill the glycogen reserves. Your athletes cannot build up their glycogen stores in a few short hours before a match or event because, as muscle biopsy research studies have documented, it takes 2-3 days to restore depleted muscle glycogen levels. It is for this reason that crash dieting is such an ineffective weight loss technique. The food deprivation or starvation tactics used in crash dieting mean that the athlete will be eating considerably smaller quantities of carbohydrates than usual. Thus, the muscles will not have their normal supply of glycogen, which could impair muscle function. Numerous tests by researchers clearly demonstrate that food deprivation reduces muscle glycogen stores; therefore, the longer the activity or event in which athletes participate, the more severe the effect on muscle performance. In other words, the athlete who has been crash dieting runs the risk of running out of fuel for the muscles during competition, and this fuel cannot be replaced by eating candy bars or even pasta a few hours before the game or event.

The contribution of liver glycogen also should not be overlooked. Insulin allows the liver as well as muscle to store glucose as glycogen.

The significance of this liver glycogen becomes apparent when one realizes that nerve cells, particularly those in the brain, are dependent upon blood glucose for their fuel supply. Nerve cells do not store glucose and they do not readily use fat as a fuel. Thus, it is critical that blood glucose levels be maintained because without a continual supply of blood glucose, the nerve tissue of the brain would be unable to function. Those who have ever missed a couple of meals have experienced some effects of decreased glucose supplies to the brain. When the brain's cells are deprived of their optimal fuel supply, they do not function well. Consequently, in addition to feeling hungry, we are unable to concentrate and we become lethargic.

After a meal containing carbohydrates, the blood glucose is readily available to the brain; several hours later, however, the blood glucose level begins to decrease because glucose is being taken out by the muscles as well as the brain. At this point, the liver glycogen becomes important. The liver can turn glycogen back into glucose and release it into the blood, thereby maintaining blood glucose levels for the brain's use. The decreasing blood glucose level not only signals the liver to release glucose, but it also signals the pancreas to stop releasing insulin. Because all cells except nerve cells need insulin to use glucose, stopping the release of insulin is the body's way of ensuring that only the nerve cells may use the blood glucose.

Because athletes and other performers must feel energetic, must be able to concentrate, and must be able to have their nerves control thousands of muscle contractions, they can ill-afford to have inade-

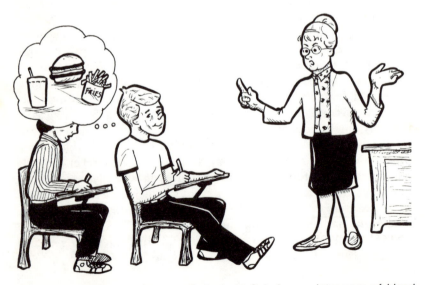

Figure 4.2. *Without adequate carbohydrate Calories, maintenance of blood glucose concentration is impossible.*

quate liver glycogen levels. Instead of crash dieting, athletes should be trying to optimize their liver glycogen levels. Let's find out how they can do so.

Are All Carbohydrates Equally Good Glucose Sources?

During training, athletes can best maintain adequate glycogen levels by consuming 50-55% of their calories in the form of complex carbohydrates, such as those listed in Table 4.1. These carbohydrates contain fiber and bulk, which are necessary for the health of the gastrointestinal tract. Diets that are low in bulk and fiber are thought to be related to cancer of the colon and other intestinal diseases. Furthermore, complex carbohydrates are digested somewhat more slowly than are simple carbohydrates such as those found in cakes, pies, cookies, and candy. This means that the glucose will be released more slowly and *evenly* into the blood stream, as shown in Figure 4.3. Consequently, less insulin will be released. When junk foods containing simple sugars are eaten, the blood glucose level shoots up, resulting in a "carbohydrate high." The large quantities of insulin that are released, however, cause the blood glucose level to plunge. This causes the individual to "crash" from the carbohydrate high, resulting in temporary hypoglycemia. No one, particularly an athlete, can afford these wild fluctuations in the blood sugar levels, for they have adverse effects on the nervous system. Furthermore, these types of junk foods can lead to vitamin deficiencies, as pointed out in chapter 3. Thus, all the facts lead to one conclusion: Athletes should avoid junk foods, especially during training.

Not all complex carbohydrates are the best source of carbohydrates immediately before competition. Some complex carbohydrates are inappropriate because they have a lot of bulk which takes a long time to

Table 4.1

Sources of Complex Carbohydrates

Fresh and dried fruits	Whole-grain bread
Potatoes	Whole wheat crackers
Sweet potatoes	Cornflakes, granola, Grapenuts,
Pasta	Shredded Wheat, Cheerios
Fresh vegetables	Whole-grain cookies and cakes
Vegetables	Tortillas

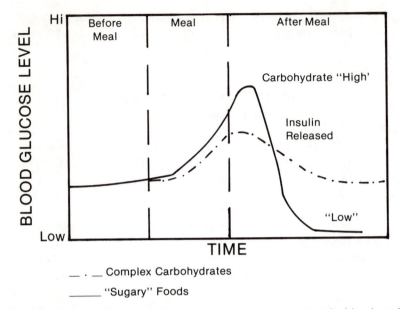

Figure 4.3. *The rapid release of large quantities of glucose into the blood, such as occurs after eating candy, is also followed by a plunge in blood glucose, resulting in a "carbohydrate high" followed by a low or down period.*

digest and which consequently slows athletes down. Thus, athletes should avoid high fiber, high bulk carbohydrates before competing. Sherbets, fruit juices, and low bulk fruits such as those listed in Table 4.2 are particularly delicious ways to "top off" glycogen stores with low fiber, easily digested carbohydrates. The old stand-by, chocolate candy bars, are not good sources of quick energy and should be avoided because the chocolate contains both fats and caffeine. The fat slows down digestion and caffeine can increase nervousness and jitters in an already excited athlete.

As part of your athletes' nutritional education, take some time to explain what carbohydrates are and why complex carbohydrates are far superior to the simple sugar found in junk foods. In fact, try it yourself and see if you don't feel better and have a more consistent energy level.

Even though maximal performance is impossible without muscle glycogen, carbohydrates are not the only fuel food. Fats are equally important.

Fats

Contrary to some popular myths in the sports world, fats are an im-

Table 4.2

Low Residue, Nutritious Carbohydrate Sources

Tapioca pudding	Shakes made with sherbets and
Puddings and gelatin desserts	fruit drinks
Fruit juices	Potatoes without skin
Graham crackers, angel food	(baked or boiled)
cake, and sponge cake	Cooked pureed vegetables, such
Bananas and avocados	as asparagus, beets, carrots,
Sherberts and ice milk	peas, pumpkin, and squash
Cooked or canned apples,	Hy-Cal®
apricots, cherries, peaches,	Cal-Power®
and pears	

portant energy source. They also are needed for building cell membranes, skin, hormones, and other structural and functional components of the body. Although they do not provide energy as quickly as do carbohydrates, more energy can be stored as fats. Thus, fats provide important fuel sources for prolonged activities. In fact, recent research with marathon runners has revealed that performance can be substantially improved if fats can be mobilized and used as a fuel early in the race so that the body's glycogen stores can be saved for later.

Furthermore, fats are a good source of high-density Calories. One gram of carbohydrate contains water plus 4 Calories of energy, whereas 1 gram of fat contains less water and about 9 Calories of energy. But not all fats are equally valuable as calorie sources. Those fats which are derived from animal sources have a high percentage of saturated fats, which have all possible sites for hydrogen molecules filled with hydrogen molecules. Fats derived from plant sources, however, are unsaturated, which means that some of the hydrogen sites are unfilled. Diets high in saturated or animal fats are thought to lead to increased incidences of atherosclerosis and cardiovascular disease. Therefore, the American Heart Association has strongly recommended that we reduce the amount of saturated fat in our diet.

What this means to the coach is that athletes should be encouraged to include fats (20-30% of the Calories) in their meals in order to obtain the proper balance of nutrients. Coaches should also emphasize that vegetable oils and plant fat sources are best. Particular care should be taken to convey the dangers associated with high saturated fat diets to athletes involved in weight gain programs. Eating high saturated fats not only negates the success of a weight gain program, but it also fosters poor lifetime eating habits.

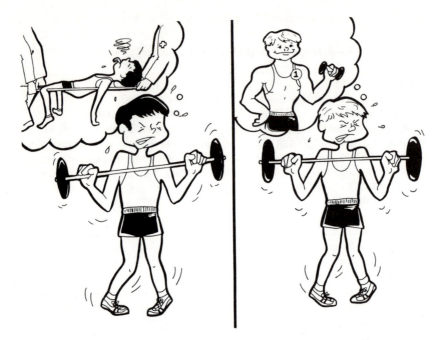

Figure 4.4. *Athletes' self-confidence is affected by what they do and don't eat. If their body is suffering from a crash diet, their self-concept is likely to suffer as well.*

The Dangers of High-Fat, High-Protein Diets

You need to be aware that athletes on high-fat, high-protein diets, whether they are losing or gaining weight or depleting glycogen stores as part of the High Octane Diet plan (see chapter 10), will not be able to work as hard or perform as well as usual. They simply do not have the fuel—glycogen—to do so; stored fat and body proteins will be their fuels. Because fat cannot be "burned" completely without glycogen, excess fat is left in the body, which causes the body to produce ketones. These substances are acid in nature and disturb the body's acid-base balance. A high-fat, high-protein diet also challenges the body's water balance because of the body proteins which must be broken down. Then the kidneys will have to excrete excess water to remove the protein by-product uric acid (see chapters 1 and 5). Such a situation may be tolerable as part of the High Octane Diet Plan because this is done only on rare occasions, but the repeated or long-term use of high-protein, high-fat diets for weight control or other purposes has NO PLACE in the world of sport. Not only is the body's energy production potential hampered, but the athlete's psychological state may be disrupted as well.

It was readily apparent from the account of Davey's experience in chapter 1 that "making weight" was not the best thing for his ego or self-concept. Anyone demonstrating such symptoms of depression is not reflecting a healthy self-concept. The wrestler who feels too weak to win is in trouble. If these feelings persist and are strong enough, an athlete may develop a "loser's complex." Obviously, youngsters who have a positive view of their physical selves and physical accomplishments are much more likely to be able to carry this view over into other spheres of their lives. Self-confidence also is likely to suffer if the young athlete's academic performance in school suffers as a result of crash diets. The athlete's ability to concentrate is particularly vulnerable to these stresses and strains.

In addition to its potential impact upon the psychological outlook of athletes, high-fat, high-protein diets as well as crash dieting practices also can take their toll on athletes' relationships with others. For example, some athletes may be withdrawn, and sometimes even bitter, during rapid weight loss conditions. They may behave completely unlike their usual self. They may be irritable and brusque, causing hard feelings on the part of their family and friends. These youngsters usually aren't aware of the negative feelings they are causing because they assume that everyone must understand the agony they are going through. Although athletes are actually glad someone cares, they may

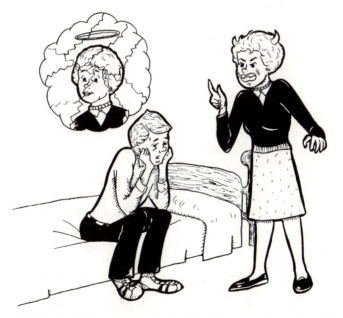

Figure 4.5. *Crash dieters frequently feel that their loved ones have "turned on them."*

frequently complain that they wish everyone would just "get off their back."

Athletes who behave this way while on a crash diet have some legitimate reasons for doing so. In order for the brain to function properly, millions and millions of chemical reactions must occur. Because the optimal rate of these chemical reactions depends upon the availability of water, dehydration can directly impair the function of the brain. The dehydrated athlete literally cannot think or concentrate as well as usual.

The body also has a biological response to food deprivation in that it has a built-in safety mechanism for those circumstances in which food is not readily available. As discussed earlier, when carbohydrates are available in the intestine, glucose is absorbed from the intestine into the blood. Then insulin allows glucose to be used and the extra glucose to be stored in muscle cells and the liver. Once all of the carbohydrates from a meal are digested, glucose no longer enters the blood from the intestine. Thus, as the cells of the body continue to use blood glucose for fuel, the blood glucose level falls. Remember, however, that the nerve cells are dependent upon glucose as a fuel because nerve cells do not readily "burn" fat as fuel. Furthermore, nerve cells do not store glucose, so they are very dependent upon a continuous supply of blood glucose. To ensure that adequate glucose is available to the brain, the body will set a number of chemical reactions into operation. Specifically, when the blood glucose level drops to a critical point, the body releases several hormones (epinephrine, known as adrenaline, is a major one of these hormones). These hormones cause the following reactions:

1. The liver releases its stored glucose into the blood.

2. The muscles start using their glycogen stores.

3. Fat is released from storage so it can be used as a fuel.

4. Body proteins are broken down so the liver can use the resultant amino acids to make glucose.

Although this elaborate and ingenious set of reactions helps the brain maintain a fuel supply, the very same hormones that control these reactions also influence how we feel. These hormones are responsible for the nervous, jumpy, irritable feelings that we experience after skipping a meal or two. So, the very hormones that are released to maintain blood glucose levels can actually change behavior!

Summary

The information in this chapter should help you to better understand how the body utilizes fuel foods, making it easier to promote appropriate eating strategies for your athletes. In addition, you should now be able to understand the behavior patterns you've seen among athletes and to recognize the symptoms of crash dieting and low blood sugar levels.

Chapter 5
Water, Water Everywhere

Water is just as necessary for good nutrition as carbohydrates, fats, proteins, vitamins, and minerals. Unfortunately, many athletes do not realize this and use water restriction and water loss to lose weight rapidly. Water is vital during performance, something you and your athletes must understand. In addition, you and your athletes should also be aware of the circumstances which influence the body's water content. In this chapter, you will learn about water—what it is, what it does, and why it is so important.

Water: What Is It?

Water is a simple compound comprised of two atoms of hydrogen and one oxygen, as shown in the formula: H_2O. It is not only essential for optimal physical performance but for life. In such sports as wrestling, sometimes athletes are more concerned about "making weight" than the value of water to their performance. Because water weighs about 1 lb per pint, the body's weight can be reduced dramatically by limiting fluid consumption and stimulating water losses. The ramifications of water restriction can be severe, however.

Is Water Weight Excess Weight?

Healthy youngsters' weight is 45 to 65% water. Although this may sound like a lot, none of the water is excess. To explain why, let's examine where this water is located and how it contributes to life processes.

Water is distributed in a number of different compartments or spaces within the body. The extracellular compartment, as shown in Figure 5.1, consists of all of those "spaces" in the body which are located outside the cells and which contain water. Blood plasma, for instance, which is primarily comprised of water, represents one of the extracellular fluid compartments and constitutes about 5% of the body's weight. Some extracellular water is also found in the hollow organs, the joints, and in bones, but the greatest quantity of extracel-

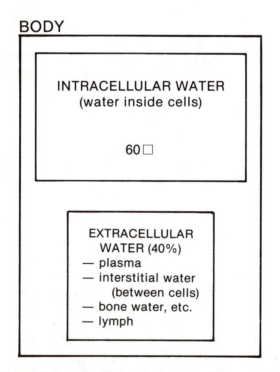

Figure 5.1. *The body has two major water compartments. The intracellular compartment represents the water held inside the cells of the body, whereas the extracellular water represents water found outside cells in such places as the blood plasma, lymph, and cerebral spinal fluid.*

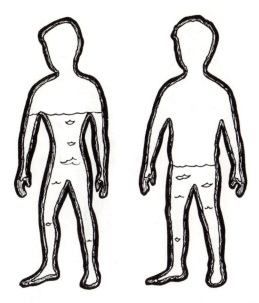

Figure 5.2. *Muscle cells contain more water than do fat cells; therefore, the individual with more body fat will have less body water than will a well-conditioned athlete.*

lular fluid—the intercellular fluid—surrounds and bathes the cells. The largest amount of water, however, is located inside the body's cells (intracellular fluid). The muscle cells in particular contain a great deal of water, so much so that 70% of their weight is from water. On the other hand, fat contains much less water.

This means that the lean, well-trained athlete, shown on the left in Figure 5.2, has more body water than does his nonathlete classmate who has more body fat. This DOES NOT mean, however, that the athlete can afford to lose more water weight. Participants in high energy output and endurance activities especially need adequate levels of body water. For example, a Swiss team's unsuccessful attempt to climb Mount Everest was attributed to their small supply of water. They had brought only sufficient fuel to melt snow for 1 pint a day per man during the ascent. As the climbers became dehydrated, fatigue developed and forced them to turn back. A later climbing party was successful, but they carried enough fuel to provide each man with 7 pints of water per day!

Perhaps the athlete's need for body water can best be understood by briefly examining the functions of water in the body, especially as they relate to physical activity. Water is essential because it:

1. serves as a solvent,

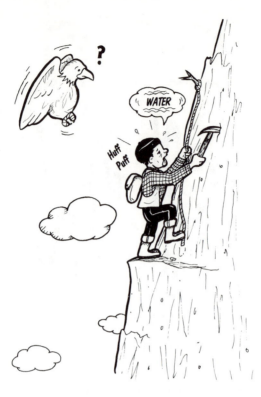

Figure 5.3. *Adequate water is essential to prevent fatigue and allow for optimal muscular function.*

2. aids in the body's temperature regulation processes, and

3. serves as a medium for chemical reactions.

Water as a Solvent

Because water is a medium compatible with many compounds, it serves as an excellent means of transporting substances. For example, various nutrients, hormones, and even antibodies are transported in the water of the blood plasma to the intercellular fluid, the water which surrounds the individual cells. Likewise, the waste products released by the cells are carried away by water. Without such a highly efficient transport mechanism, the nourishment of the cells would be impossible.

Water as a Temperature Regulator

Water has two major roles to play in the process of regulating the

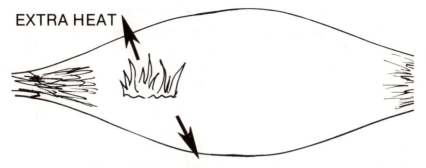

EXTRA HEAT

ENERGY FOR CONTRACTION

Figure 5.4. *As the body's cells, including the muscle cells, burn fuel to release energy for life maintenance as well as movement, a great deal of excess heat energy is given off.*

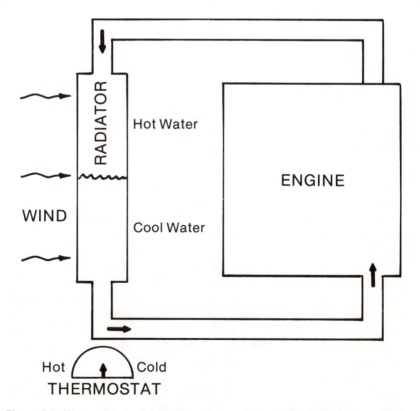

Figure 5.5. *Water aids in the cooling of most automobile engines because it picks up a heat load and carries this to the radiator where the heat escapes and the water temperature drops so that the process can start over.*

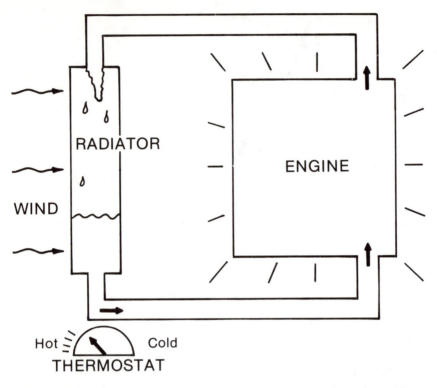

Figure 5.6. *If the water level in the car's radiator becomes low, the cooling system no longer works. Similarly, if the blood plasma level becomes too low, as in dehydration, one of the body's major cooling systems no longer works.*

body's temperature. First of all, water can absorb a considerable amount of heat before its temperature rises. Even while at rest, each of the cells of the body is continually burning fuels to provide energy for life processes (see Figure 5.4). A large portion of the released energy is not useful energy; rather, it is heat energy. During physical activity, the body's energy need increases, and thus, the rate at which fuel is burned increases accordingly. In other words, the cells of the body are similar to the combustion engines in cars. As these engines burn gasoline, energy is released to propel the car, but a considerable amount of energy is also given off as heat. Automobiles have cooling systems to prevent the engines from overheating, as shown in Figure 5.5. Similarly, if the heat given off by the muscle cells and the other cells of the body is not dispelled from the body, the body temperature soars, destroying structural proteins as well as the enzymes which regulate the various chemical reactions in the body.

Because each tissue is made up of thousands of layers of cells, dissipating the heat directly into the environment would be too slow a

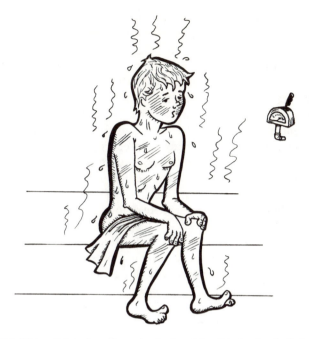

Figure 5.7. *This athlete is unknowingly depriving his body of vital water.*

process. Thus, the intercellular water that bathes the cells and the circulating blood plasma works much like the water cooling system which cools your car engine. The plasma picks up the heat and carries it to the skin's surface, where the heat escapes into the environment. If the heart were not continually pumping blood to circulate the plasma in order to absorb heat from the cells, and if water could not absorb such large quantities of heat so readily, it would be very difficult for the body to cool itself.

This ingenious cooling system, however, is only able to work efficiently if the blood volume and intracellular fluid volume are adequate. Just as the car's engine in Figure 5.6 will overheat if the radiator's water level is low, so too will the body's cooling system fail if the volume of circulating water (blood and intracellular fluid) is decreased. This is exactly what happens when athletes choose to lose weight by losing water or dehydrating. Sweating in steam rooms, using water pills, and any other procedures designed to lose weight quickly by dehydrating will result in a reduced efficiency of the circulatory system, one of the body's major cooling systems.

Despite the efficiency of the circulating cooling system, in hot climates and during strenuous exercise, the circulating blood cannot keep pace with the need to dissipate heat. At this point, the second major heat-regulating contribution of water comes into play: sweat.

Contrary to popular belief, however, it is not the actual act of sweating which does the cooling; it is the *evaporation* of the water in the sweat. It takes energy for water to be changed from its liquid form to its gas form: water vapor. If you place water in a pan and place the pan in a room, the water evaporates slowly. If, however, you place the pan on the stove and add heat energy, the water molecules speed up their movements and escape more quickly, hastening the evaporation process. Heat from the body does precisely the same thing to the water molecules in the sweat. The body heat energy supplies the necessary energy to speed up evaporation, and in doing so, heat is lost from the body as water molecules escape to become water vapor.

Water as a Medium for Chemical Reactions

Even though the excess heat energy produced by the chemical reactions taking place in the cells sometimes poses a cooling problem for the body, life would be impossible if those chemical reactions ceased. These chemical reactions are necessary to release the needed energy

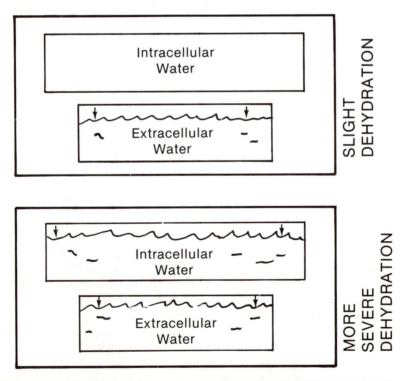

Figure 5.8. *During the initial stages of dehydration, water is first lost from the plasma and interstitial fluid (extracellular spaces), and then as the dehydration progresses water is lost from the cells themselves (intracellular water).*

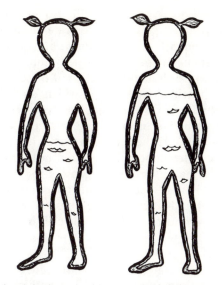

Figure 5.9. *While the dehydrated athlete on the left has a lower scale weight than the athlete on the right, this athlete has deprived the chemical engines in her muscles of their required water.*

for life functions, and water is the medium in which these reactions take place. In fact, the higher the reaction rate or metabolic rate within a cell, the greater will be that cell's water content. This is the reason why muscle or lean tissue has a higher water content than does fat tissue; more water is required to carry out the chemical reactions involved in the vigorous functions of the muscle.

The needed water will not be available in the muscles or other cells if athletes lose weight by losing water. For not only do dehydrating tactics take water from the blood plasma and other extracellular spaces, they also draw water from the cells themselves (see Figure 5.8). These cells, due to their diminished water volume, also will have a diminished capacity to produce energy.

Thus, water is an important quantity for efficient body function, especially for athletes who participate in daily, energy-demanding, practice sessions. Even though a large percent of their body weight is comprised of water, these athletes can ill afford to jeopardize their body hydration levels.

Why Is It Potentially Hazardous for the Athlete to Dehydrate?

Each of the functions of water we have mentioned is critical not only to wrestlers if they are to give their "all" on the mat, but are equally important to ice skaters trying to concentrate on the maneuvers of an intricate routine, gymnasts who train long hours, and football players who need the stamina to perform in hot, humid weather. For the heart, lungs, and entire circulatory system of these athletes to be functioning optimally, their blood volume, which is 45-50% water, must be adequate. Dehydration is the loss of body water from the various body fluid compartments including plasma, the water bathing the cells, and the water inside the cells. The reduction of plasma, for example, thus reduces the blood volume. This means that the heart must pump much faster than usual to compensate for the reduced volume of blood, for the blood is faced with the relentless tasks of transporting oxygen and fuel to the "engine-like" muscle cells as well as removing wastes and by-products. If the muscle cells do not receive enough oxygen and fuel, they will not be able to produce the energy athletes need.

Scientists have investigated the effects of reduced availability of oxygen during dehydration by first dehydrating athletes and then having them perform various types of hard physical exercise. During these hard workouts, such as running on a treadmill, a special mouth piece is used to collect air and determine how much oxygen has been used (oxygen consumption), as illustrated in Figure 5.10. Then, after

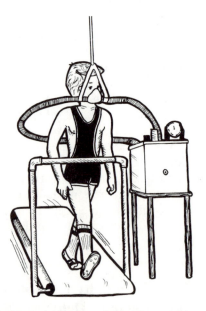

Figure 5.10. *Treadmills and other special testing equipment have been used to determine how dehydration influences the ability of the muscle to use oxygen in order to burn fuel.*

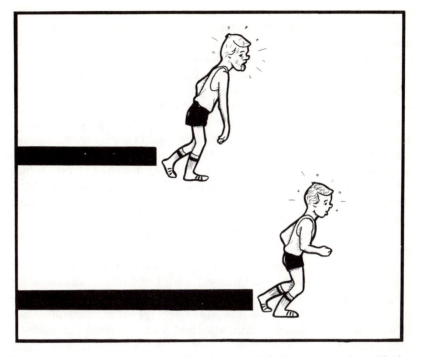

Figure 5.11. *Athletes who begin exercise in a dehydrated state (as with the athlete on the top) will not be able to work as long as athletes who begin with normal hydration (like the athlete on the bottom).*

recovering and rehydrating, the athlete repeats the same experiment. Again, the maximum amount of work and the maximum oxygen consumption are recorded. The results led scientists to conclude that while dehydration probably does not reduce the capacity to consume a maximal amount of oxygen, it does reduce the amount of time an athlete can work hard before being exhausted. These same studies also indicated that even the heart of a dehydrated athlete working below his or her maximum must do more work than it would have to do under normal conditions.

In addition to carrying oxygen, the blood's role in heat removal is particularly important. If this heat is allowed to build, the resultant tissue and enzyme destruction can be lethal. So it is vital that the body fluid volumes are not diminished by dehydration.

Furthermore, as the extracellular water is lost during dehydration, water is actually drawn from the cells because the body attempts to balance the water concentration inside and outside of the cells. Thus, the cells, especially the muscle cells, will have less water available to support their energy-producing chemical reactions. It is these very chemical reactions which are necessary to supply the energy for performing well in sports.

Perhaps you are thinking, "But I've seen athletes perform well after dehydrating." True, the energy-producing machinery does not grind to a halt, but neither is it functioning optimally. Do you want your athletes to play when their energy-production system is below par?

Still another deleterious effect of decreasing the body's fluid volume is the impact on kidney function. Normally, the kidney may filter as many as 180 liters of plasma a day (a liter is slightly more than a quart). Most of the filtered plasma gets back into the blood, because the kidney produces only 1 to 1.5 liters of urine daily. This filtration of large quantities of plasma, however, is not a wasted effort. While filtering the plasma, the kidney removes liquid wastes and regulates electrolyte levels (see chapter 6). In fact, the filtration of a certain quantity of plasma is essential if the kidney itself is to remain healthy. If sufficient plasma is not available for filtration, the kidney can sustain serious damage.

Medical authorities have, therefore, advised that urine production should not be allowed to fall below 1200 ml and this urine should be clear and colorless, rather than yellow and concentrated. Urine production below this quantity is quite likely for the athlete employing rapid weight loss tactics because the fluid restriction and dehydration practices characteristic of rapid weight loss decrease the flow of blood through the kidney (renal flow), resulting in a decreased volume of fluid filtered by the kidney. Not only may rapid weight loss techniques detract from the athlete's performance, the use of these techniques may be detrimental for a vital organ: the kidney.

Up to this point, we have talked about the effects of dehydration in a rather general way. An examination of specific dehydrating techniques reveals still more reasons why you need to implement steps to keep your athletes from dehydrating themselves.

Dehydration Techniques

As has been noted previously, the body's water content is divided into a number of different compartments, as can be seen in Figure 5.1. In addition, the volume of the water varies from compartment to compartment and the water losses from the various compartments can be disproportionate. For example, the dehydration stemming from excessive sweating will decrease the extracellular water first. Then if the dehydration process continues, water will be drawn out of the cells themselves (see Figure 5.8). Many of the various dehydrating tactics will have slightly different initial effects upon the body's water compartments. These differences can best be understood by examining the various dehydrating practices athletes use. These procedures include:

- Sweating

- Induced vomiting

- Use of diuretics

- Use of cathartics

- Expectorating

For the most part, these tactics reflect exaggerations of the normal avenues for water loss. In Figure 5.12, you can see that a considerable amount of water is normally lost each day. These losses are usually offset by water consumed through either eating or drinking. Even under circumstances of only moderate temperature and light physical activity, enough water is lost that the body's entire water mass must be replaced every 11-13 days. Vigorous exercise, high temperatures, and a high relative humidity result in an even higher turnover rate. Thus, by exaggerating the avenues for water loss and restricting water replacement schedules, athletes have used dehydration as a means of "making weight"—either for specific competitions as in wrestling and

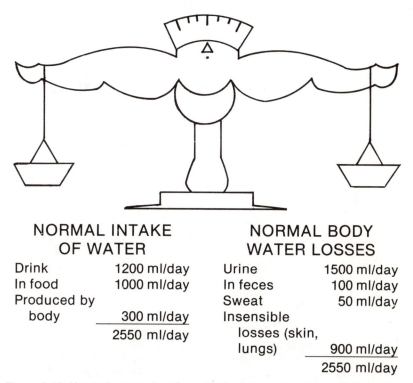

NORMAL INTAKE OF WATER		NORMAL BODY WATER LOSSES	
Drink	1200 ml/day	Urine	1500 ml/day
In food	1000 ml/day	In feces	100 ml/day
Produced by body	300 ml/day	Sweat	50 ml/day
	2550 ml/day	Insensible losses (skin, lungs)	900 ml/day
			2550 ml/day

Figure 5.12. Normally water lost from the body is replaced on a daily basis.

crew or just as a means of maintaining their body weights.

We have already described the general dangers of dehydration, but now we will discuss the various dehydrating tactics and their specific effects on the body.

Dehydration Via Sweating

Sweat, the fluid secreted by the sweat glands, contains extracellular water along with small quantities of "salts" (electrolytes). Because the evaporation of sweat provides a means of losing body heat, the onset of sweating is controlled by a thermostat in the brain called the hypothalamus. Thus, the thermostat detects when body temperature rises above a specified level, causing sweating to begin and continue until body temperature is reduced or the body's water content is too low to support further sweating. The athlete can therefore reduce body weight significantly by stimulating the sweating mechanism.

This of course can be accomplished by engaging in physical activity, or being in a hot room (thermal stress), or a combination of both.

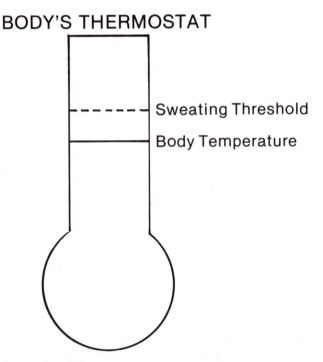

BODY'S THERMOSTAT

------- Sweating Threshold

Body Temperature

Figure 5.13. *The hypothalamus, a brain center, contains the body's thermostat. When the body temperature reaches a specified point, sweating begins and will continue as long as the temperature remains elevated and the body has ample water.*

Thermal stress may further exaggerate water loss from physical activity because it prevents evaporation, resulting in greater sweating. This happens because without evaporation the body temperature will stay elevated and the brain's thermostat will continue to stimulate the sweating mechanism.

Increasing the relative humidity of an environment can stop evaporation. Therefore, standing in a hot shower or steam room, or sitting in a hot bath will elevate body temperature and stimulate sweating. The sweat, however, cannot evaporate, allowing little or no cooling effect, so the profuse sweating continues.

When using physical activity as a means of inducing sweating, an individual uses some of the energy released from the fuel foods for the activity and the excess energy builds up as heat in the body, raising the body temperature. When the body temperature reaches the specified level, the hypothalamus initiates sweating. If the sweat evaporates, the skin is cooled and body heat can escape, preventing the body temperature from going too high. The more exercise that is done, the larger the volume of sweat that is lost. Exaggeration of water loss through exercise is accomplished by preventing the evaporation of the sweat and the escape of body heat. This procedure is really a combination of thermal stress and exercise stress. By wearing excessive layers of clothing or by increasing the room temperature, the individual is using thermal stress to further stimulate the exercise-induced sweating. Furthermore, the excessive clothing impairs the evaporation of sweat from the skin. This is particularly true if rubberized clothing is worn.

Tremendous quantities of water can be lost in this fashion, about 2-3 liters per hour up to a maximum of 12 liters. In fact, on hot, humid days, up to 20 lbs of water loss have been recorded for some large athletes. Of course, losses of this magnitude seriously jeopardize health; and all too frequently, they can result in death due to decreases in blood, which impairs the body's cooling mechanisms. But even less drastic levels of dehydration have been shown to hinder performance. Nonetheless, sweat-induced dehydration is a common practice in certain sports.

Thermal stress can also be dangerous in another way. In response to the heat, blood vessels all over the body's surface dilate or open up. This allows blood to pass through vessels which are close to the surface, thus making it easier for the "heat load" to move from the warm blood to a relatively cooler environment. This dilation explains why skin becomes red as the body temperature rises. The red coloration indicates that the blood is merely flowing closer to the surface. If the athlete is submerged in hot water or sitting in a sauna, vessels dilate all over the body. It takes a lot of blood to fill all of these vessels. Consequently, the amount of blood flowing to the brain is reduced. The re-

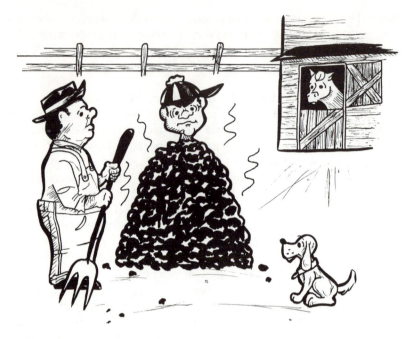

Figure 5.14. *Athletes have been very creative in constructing "sweat boxes" for weight loss.*

sult is drowsiness or even unconsciousness. For this reason, trainers must never leave athletes unattended in hot, whole-body whirlpools: an athlete could easily nod off to sleep and slip under the water and drown. All too frequently, the reducing athlete is alone in the steam room, shower, or bathtub. In fact, there have been tragic reports of fatalities from young athletes passing out and drowning or passing out and dying from head injuries under these conditions. So the threat of danger from both the direct and indirect use of thermal stress is real indeed.

The preceding physiological review of the ills of rapid weight loss will help you better understand the concern of the American College of Sports Medicine. . . a concern which prompted them to publish position papers on weight loss in wrestling and water needs for distance running. These position papers are reproduced in Appendices E and F. Although the position statements directly address wrestlers and runners, the contents are applicable to other athletes.

Dehydration Via Vomiting

The food we eat goes from the mouth into the stomach rather quickly, but it is some time before the food is digested and the various

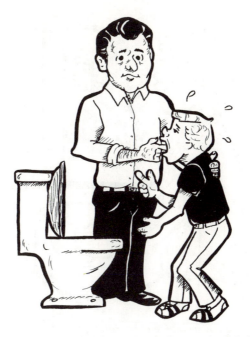

Figure 5.15. *Some reports claim that parents have taken their youngster's weight control into their own hands.*

nutrients are absorbed through the intestinal wall. Consequently, some athletes, as well as the parents of young athletes, have taken advantage of this time delay between eating and absorption. These athletes allow themselves to experience all of the pleasurable experiences associated with eating, but before the food can be moved out of the stomach, a finger or other noxious object is used to induce vomiting. Thus, all of the calorie-containing food is ejected from the stomach. In reality, much more than just food has been ejected. Large quantities of water and chloride, in the form of hydrochloric acid, and other fluids are excreted by the glands in the walls of the stomach to aid in the digestive processes. Usually these fluids and other substances would be absorbed in the large intestine, and therefore, not lost from the body. Vomiting, however, results in the loss of large quantities of water and electrolytes as well as the original food. True, these losses do help to reduce the body's weight, but at the expense of body water. In addition to dehydrating the athlete, forced vomiting also causes serious destruction of the body's salt or electrolyte balances (see chapter 6).

The hydrochloric acid from the stomach can also "burn" the esophagus, mouth, and lips of the athlete. Furthermore, the loss of acid disturbs the body's acid-base balance, adding yet another

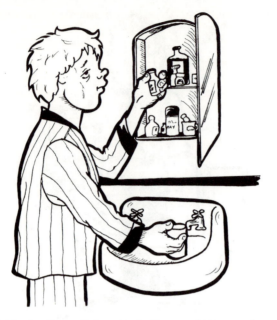

Figure 5.16. *The family medicine chest often provides a ready source of water pills.*

obstacle to the efficiency of the muscle's energy-producing chemical reactions.

Dehydration Via "Water Pills"

The kidney continually filters plasma from the blood, removing waste products and then returning most of the plasma to the blood. The wastes and plasma water which remain in the kidney are then excreted from the body as urine. The actual volume of urine excreted is under the control of hormones. Thus, by regulating the levels of these various hormones, the quantity of urine that is produced and excreted can be regulated. The so-called "water pill" is really a diuretic or a substance which prevents much of the plasma water filtered by the kidney from being returned to the blood. Thus, more than the normal quantity of urine is excreted. Several pounds of weight can be lost by taking water pills, but only at the expense of the body's critical water supply.

Similarly, diuretic effects can also be realized by consuming beverages containing caffeine, such as coffee, tea, certain cola drinks, and cocoa rather than actually taking water pills. Emotional pressure and nervousness also tend to have diuretic effects, which could further compound dehydration and detract from athletic performance potential.

Dehydration Via Laxatives

As discussed previously, large amounts of fluid are secreted into the food by the glands in the walls of the stomach and still more fluids are secreted in the intestine. Normally, the water in this fluid is not lost to the body because 99% of it is usually reabsorbed in the large intestine. As can be seen in Figure 5.12, only 3-5% of the daily water loss occurs through the feces. This picture changes dramatically if laxatives or cathartics are taken. These products stimulate the wall of the large intestine to eject wastes before the water can be absorbed. Consequently, substantial quantities of body water can be lost in this manner. In addition, not only are the body's water compartments being depleted, but substantial potassium and other electrolyte losses occur.

Similarly, athletes who suffer with a bout of diarrhea are left with a weak, washed-out feeling. Athletes cannot afford to lose these fluids and electrolytes—either voluntarily by taking laxatives or involuntarily through a case of diarrhea!

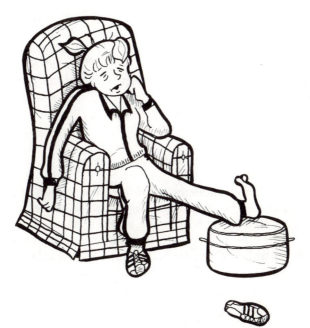

Figure 5.17. *Because laxatives drain athletes' body water and electrolytes, they leave athletes with a weak, washed-out feeling.*

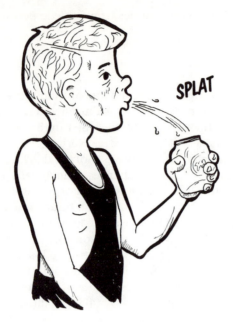

Figure 5.18. *Expectoration is just another way athletes rid themselves of necessary body water.*

Dehydration Via Expectoration

The sight of wrestlers spitting into cups is not uncommon, as this technique is used as a last effort to cut weight. The saliva or "spit" is manufactured by salivary glands. Water is the primary constituent, thus repeated spitting or expectoration constitutes another drain on the body's critical water supply.

Summary

For lean, conditioned athletes, a considerable portion of their body weight is water weight, but this water weight is not excess weight. Water plays a significant role in the functioning of the body, and therefore, the healthy athlete really does not have water to spare. This is why later chapters will repeatedly stress that the establishment of good water-drinking habits is fundamental to sound nutritional conditioning programs.

Chapter 6
Electro-What's?

Along with understanding the vital role of water, you should understand what electrolytes are and what roles they play in body function. We used the term *electrolyte* when discussing water balance but we did not explain what an electrolyte is or why they are necessary. Let's do so now.

What is an Electrolyte?

An electrolyte is not a new wonder drug which scientists have just discovered, nor is it a miracle food additive which assures athletic prowess. Rather, an electrolyte is a "charged" molecule. Normally, most molecules are neutral. That is, they have an equal number of positive protons and negative electrons. Salt, for instance, is chemically represented by the symbol NaCl, with the Na standing for sodium and the Cl for chloride. Thus, sodium chloride does not have an electrical charge, but when placed in water, the sodium and chloride separate, producing two electrolytes—

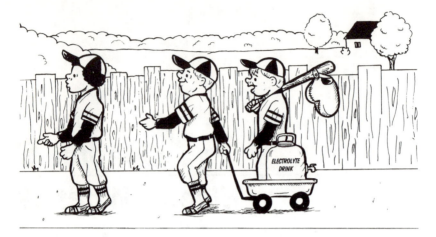

Figure 6.1. *Although athletes at all levels are beginning to use electrolyte drinks, many athletes as well as coaches do not understand the functions of electrolytes.*

Na^+ and Cl^-. These charged molecules have an important role to play in various life functions (see Figure 6.2), so it is absolutely essential that the body maintain the appropriate quantities of the various electrolytes.

Maintaining the appropriate quantities of electrolytes is an on-going process because the body can lose electrolytes through several pathways. The body's electrolyte supply must be continually replenished by a diet that includes fruits, vegetables, and meats. These foods provide the necessary electrolytes (Sodium = Na^+; Potassium = K^+; Chloride = Cl^-; Calcium = Ca^+; Hydrogen = H^+). Once ingested, electrolytes can be found in a number of locations

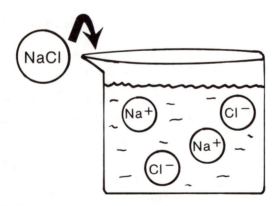

Figure 6.2. *When salt (NaCl) is placed in water, it separates into two electrolytes: Na^+ and Cl^-.*

Table 6.1

Distribution of Various Electrolytes
in the Body's Fluid Compartments

Electrolyte	Extracellular compartment (millimoles/liter of H_2O)	Intracellular compartment (millimoles/liter of H_2O)
Na^+	150	15
Cl^-	125	10
K^+	5	150

throughout the fluid compartments of the body. Interestingly, electrolytes do not appear in equal concentration in the different compartments. As shown in Table 6.1, sodium and potassium are found in the highest concentrations in the body fluids, but even these two electrolytes are not located in the same fluid spaces. In other words, some electrolytes are located predominantly in the extracellular fluids, whereas other electrolytes are located primarily in the intracellular fluids. For instance, higher concentrations of sodium (Na^+) are found in the extracellular fluids, whereas potassium (K^+) can be found in larger quantities inside the cells. This difference in the relative concentrations of various electrolytes is fundamental to life, because without such a balance between the inside and outside of cells, nerves would be unable to send impulses, skeletal muscles would be unable to contract, and even the heart would stop pumping.

For life functions to be carried out optimally, it is critical that the relatively large concentration of potassium inside the cell be offset or "balanced" by the sodium concentration outside the cell, as illustrated in Figure 6.3. If this balance is disturbed, body functions will deteriorate accordingly—a fate which athletes can ill afford if they wish to perform to peak capacity.

During exercise or physical work, a series of dynamic changes normally occurs in the distribution of the body's water. When the activity begins, water is immediately transferred from the extracellular fluid to the insides of the muscle cells, as illustrated in Figure 6.4. This transfer of water facilitates the energy-producing chemical reactions discussed in chapter 5 which take place in the muscle cell. The extracellular fluid that moves into the muscles is rapidly replaced by water from the blood plasma. Under normal conditions, this small decrease in the blood volume is tolerable because it plays a role in increasing the

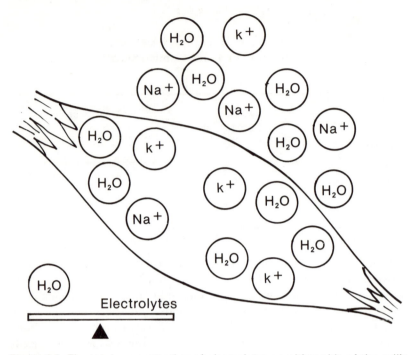

Figure 6.3. *The total concentration of electrolytes on either side of the cell's membrane must be "balanced" for life functions to continue.*

water in the cell, thus increasing the energy-production capabilities of the muscle cells.

Sodium (Salt) Imbalance

The shifting of body water into cells depends upon a delicate balance of the electrolytes in the various compartments. This is because electrolytes are not usually free to move across membranes, and therefore, water is drawn across membranes to equalize concentrations. That is, the greater the difference in the concentration of electrolytes on either side of a membrane, the greater the pressure drawing the water across the membrane to dilute the concentration of electrolytes. For example, if an excessive amount of sodium or salt (NaCl) were to be consumed, as shown in the upper half of Figure 6.5, the concentration of Na^+ in the extracellular spaces would increase. Because very little Na^+ is allowed to cross the cell membranes, the concentration of sodium in the intracellular spaces would not be altered. Thus, as a result of consuming salt, the high concentration of sodium in the extracellular spaces is larger than normal. The high con-

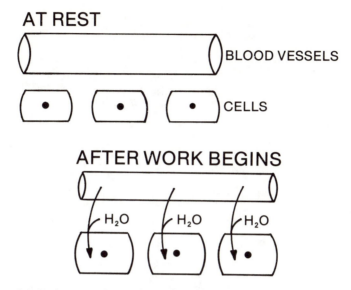

Figure 6.4. *During exercise, a characteristic shift in the body's water distribution occurs.*

centration of sodium in the extracellular spaces will draw H_2O from the intracellular compartment in order to dilute the excessive number of Na^+ ions in the extracellular space and maintain the proper concentration balance, as shown in the bottom of Figure 6.5.

Such a water shift is completed at the expense of the cell's water which, remember, is critical for the chemical reactions which produce energy. Consequently, the elevation of the sodium concentration in the extracellular fluid impairs physical performance because it prevents the shift of water into the muscle cell. This lack of cellular water results in the deterioration of that muscle's energy-production potential. Thus, the consumption of excessive salt can actually deprive the muscle cells of needed water.

The athlete who sweats excessively creates a similar situation. Sweating not only results in the loss of body water, but also disturbs the body's electrolyte balance because the sweat is primarily water, not salt (see Figure 6.6). The sweat of a well-conditioned athlete contains about 1.1 grams of Na^+ per quart of sweat, whereas the unconditioned or poorly conditioned athlete's sweat contains slightly larger quantities of Na^+ (1.8 grams/quart). In other words, the sweat is between .2% and .5% salt. Unfortunately, many coaches believe that sweat contains lots of salt and thus, that sweating results in the loss of large quantities of salt. This is not the case.

When the salt concentration in sweat is compared to the concentration of salt in the extracellular fluid, the sweat is very dilute. This

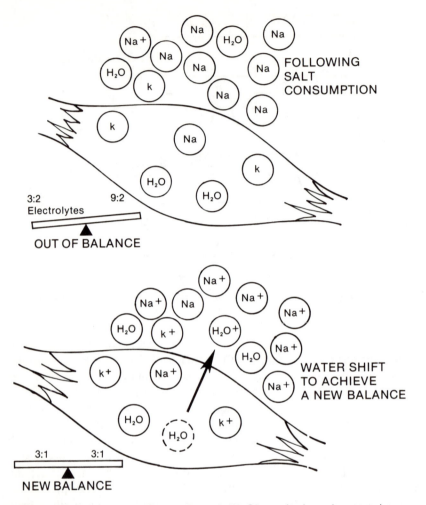

Figure 6.5. *Consumption of excessive salt (NaCl) results in an increased concentration of sodium (Na+) in the extracellular space, which draws water out of the cells to regain a concentration balance.*

means that as athletes sweat, they lose relatively more water than salt. Consequently, the fluid that is left in the extracellular spaces becomes more and more concentrated or "saltier and saltier." Again, to try and reduce this concentration, water is drawn out of the cells to dilute the extracellular fluid. And so the cell deprives itself of necessary water (see Figure 6.6).

It should be obvious how this situation frequently is made even worse by the consumption of salt tablets which are mistakenly taken to replace salt lost from sweating. Instead of helping, further concentrations of salt in the extracellular fluid disrupt the electrolyte balance

DURING EXERCISE
. . . AS SWEATING PROGRESSES

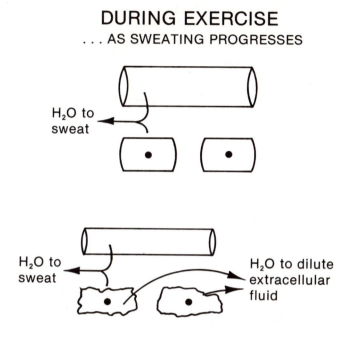

Figure 6.6. *As sweating continues during prolonged exercise, the extracellular fluid becomes more and more concentrated with sodium because the sweat contains more water than sodium (Na+). To help maintain an electrolyte balance, water is drawn from the cells, including the muscle cells, to dilute the extracellular fluid.*

by drawing needed water from the muscle cells.

It is possible to lose up to 15 grams of salt a day under extreme heat conditions, and the average daily consumption of salt is about 10 to 12 grams per day. Under these extreme conditions, some salt supplementation may be needed, but conditions are rarely this extreme. To help you with the problem of proper salt replacement, follow the schedule in Table 6.2 for salt replacement.

Consuming too much salt, then, only results in increased salt concentration in the body's extracellular fluid and the trapping of water in the extracellular spaces, which is done at the expense of the cell's water. So, when body water is available in a limited supply, as it is in the dehydrated athlete, the existing water should be made available for intracellular functions and not retained between the cells in the extracellular compartment. Obviously, then, athletes should not be encouraged to supplement their daily workouts with salt tablets unless, of course, the salt tablets are accompanied by large quantities of water.

Most authorities agree that each 7-grain salt tablet should be taken with 8 ounces of water. This helps maintain the proper electrolyte con-

Table 6.2

A Guide to Salt Replacement

Losses Due to Sweating	Replacement Need*				
Water Loss	Salt Loss				
Pounds or Pints	Grams	Grains	Water to be Replaced (Pints)	No. of 7-Grain Salt Tablets** to be Taken Per Pint of Water	
				Nonacclimatized	Acclimatized
2	1.5	23	2	0	0
4	3.0	46	4	0	0
6	4.5	69	6	0	0
8	6.0	92	8	2	1
10	7.5	115	10	4	3
12	9.0	138	12	6	5

Note. Adapted from D.K. Mathews and E.L. Fox, *The Physiological Basis of Physical Education and Athletics.* Philadelphia: W.B. Saunders, 1976.

*Because sweat contains both salt and water, both need to be replaced.

**A 7-grain salt tablet contains about ½ gram of salt.

centration. Because of the potential hazard in consuming salt tablets without adequate water, electrolyte solutions have become very popular. The consumption of these fluids ensures that adequate water intake accompanies the electrolyte consumption.

In addition to impairing physical performance, an elevated sodium concentration, or what is called hypernatermia, can impair heart function. Due to the electrolyte imbalances, the heart stays contracted; consequently, the pumping action of the heart stops and death follows. Although death can occur, a more likely outcome of too high a sodium concentration is cramping of the skeletal muscles.

The ingestion of salt tablets also can be irritating to the walls of the stomach and result in nausea. A further thought to consider is that research has shown a link between excessive salt intake and hypertension.

Further attention will be given to the topic of electrolytes and their replacement in chapters 7 and 8, when dietary guidelines for weight loss and weight gain are presented. In fact, as we point out in chapter 7, a low salt diet, rather than the consumption of salt tablets, can be a significant aid to a weight control diet.

Potassium Imbalance

So far, our discussion of electrolytes has centered on sweating and its disruption of the body's sodium balance. Na^+, however, is not the only electrolyte which may become imbalanced, nor is sweating the only means by which the body's electrolyte balances can be disturbed. In addition to sodium, human sweat also contains potassium, along with some other elements. We do not know the specific quantity of potassium lost through sweating, but apparently potassium losses in sweat are negligible under any but the most extreme conditions. Consequently, sweat-induced potassium depletion is not a primary concern and a well-balanced diet should adequately restore the potassium that is lost via sweating.

Although substantial potassium losses are not likely to occur from sweating, if cathartics or diuretics are used to effect rapid water weight losses, the drain on the body potassium can be significant. The cathartics or laxatives stimulate the early elimination of the solid waste materials in the large intestine. When solid wastes are eliminated too soon, considerable quantities of potassium and water do not have time to be absorbed and thus are lost to the body. Consequently, the use of cathartics can bring about dehydration and seriously disrupt the body's potassium levels.

Likewise, the nervous tension which frequently accompanies competition may cause neurogenic diarrhea. This type of diarrhea is the result of excessive stimulation of the parasympathetic nervous system, which greatly excites both motility of the intestine and secretion of mucus into the large intestine. These two effects can cause the rapid movement of the waste material through the large intestine, resulting in the loss of large quantities of water and potassium as well as other electrolytes.

Potassium deficiencies primarily affect the muscles and are characterized by muscular weakness which may result in paralysis. The effects of the potassium (K^+) deficiency on the smooth muscle which lines the walls of the stomach and intestine are diarrhea and intestinal distention. Such a K^+ deficiency may also cause general weakness in the heart and muscles lining the blood vessels. Obviously, then, severe potassium depletion detracts from physical performance and may even lead to death.

Similarly, forced vomiting which results in the ejection of the chyme (partially digested food) from the stomach is associated with substantial losses of water and hydrochloric acid (which contains hydrogen and chloride ions). Some sodium and potassium are also lost in this manner.

Diuretics and Electrolyte Imbalance

One of the general functions of the electrolytes is to help maintain the body's water balance. Sodium has a particularly important role to play in this regard. If the concentration of sodium falls, the kidney merely excretes water until the proper concentration of sodium and water is reestablished. The kidney will excrete water as urine only until the appropriate Na^+ concentration in the extracellular fluid has been reached. Obviously, if the kidney is stimulated to excrete extra Na^+, water also is excreted so that the concentration of Na^+ in the body fluids does not decrease.

Diuretics or "water pills" do precisely this. They effectively increase water losses by increasing the volume of urine excreted. In doing so, a diuretic must also stimulate the excretion of sodium or else the water filtered by the kidney will merely be reabsorbed into the extracellular compartment. Because chloride passively follows the sodium ion across the tubules in the kidney, any increase in the excretion of sodium by the kidney will result in a corresponding increase in the chloride ions excreted in the urine, resulting in both sodium and chloride electrolytes being out of balance. Diuretics can also disrupt the body's potassium concentration. Furthermore, the excessive urine production reduces the extracellular fluid volume so the working muscle cells are deprived of necessary water and the blood volume is diminished, forcing the heart to work harder than usual. Thus it should be clear that the "washed out," weak feeling that accompanies a seige of vomiting, or bout of diarrhea, or excessive urination, is not a psychological factor. It is a reflection of reduced blood volume and electrolyte imbalances.

Summary

Thermal stress, laxatives, diuretics, and induced vomiting can all seriously disrupt the body's electrolyte balance and fluid volume. Consequently, they have no place in the weight control practices of athletes—young or old. The unnatural regulation of body water through such tactics as water pills, laxatives, and forced vomiting is NOT the way to control weight. Specific suggestions for reducing the body's weight for optimal performance are presented next.

Chapter 7

How to Lose Weight

As you read in chapter 1, optimal body weight and physical efficiency go hand in hand. The coach who knew about body composition appraisal and sound nutritional practices was able to help his athletes enhance performance potentials. So to help you acquire these skills and knowledge, body composition appraisal and the prediction of optimal weight were discussed in chapter 2. Then to provide you with some background information about the essentials of good nutrition, chapters 3, 4, 5, and 6 discussed the various nutrients—proteins, carbohydrates, fats, vitamins, minerals, and water—and how they contribute to body function, particularly in athletes. In the next two chapters, a series of weight control guidelines will be presented to aid you in helping your athletes achieve their optimal weights. The guidelines in this chapter are for those athletes who need to lose fat to achieve their optimal percent fat, whereas chapter 8 contains some guidelines for gaining lean weight. First, however, you need to determine the optimal weights of your athletes by using the caliper technique described in chapter 2, and second, you need to understand the concept of caloric balance.

Caloric Balance

Caloric balance, the basis for the fat loss guidelines presented in this chapter, involves manipulating Calories. A Calorie or kcal is a unit of energy. Everything that we do has a caloric requirement. That is, every task requires a specific amount of energy. Even if one is lying as quietly as possible, many body functions still must take place for life to continue. These body functions use energy; the specific amount of energy can be stated in terms of Calories. Some activities require more energy and thus more Calories than other activities. On the other hand, all of the foods we eat contain a given amount of energy. Some foods contain more energy and thus more Calories than other foods.

The fact that both the energy value of foods we eat and the energy cost of your body's activities can be measured in terms of kcal, forms the basis of the concept of caloric balance. The relationship between Calories (kcal) and body weight is frequently introduced by depicting the situation in which caloric intake, the caloric content of the foods we eat, equals the caloric expenditure, the Calorie cost of our daily activities. Figure 7-1 represents this balance between caloric intake and caloric output. As long as such a balance exists and the amount of physical acitivity in your life does not change, body weight will remain constant. Remember that this body weight (as discussed in chapter 2) is comprised of fat weight and lean tissue weight. Most of the water in the body is inside the cells of the lean tissue and not the fat cells. Also, the lean tissue cells are responsible for athletic performance; they are the cells that burn fuels to provide energy for nerves to send impulses and for muscles to contract. Consequently, if young athletes are carrying around excess weight, it is in the form of fat.

Achievement of optimal physical efficiency comes with minimizing the excess *fat* weight. Fat is the important word, not just weight. Although crash dieting and dehydrating techniques can have a significant impact upon body weight, they have relatively little impact upon

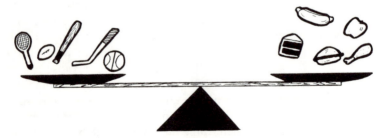

Figure 7.1. *If the body weight and body composition remain constant, the number of Calories in the food eaten will equal the number of Calories of energy expended.*

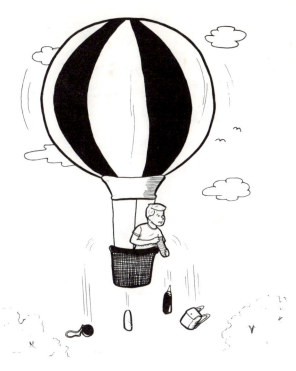

Figure 7.2. *When balloonists have to lighten the load, not all weight is considered excess weight. They cannot afford to sacrifice their burners or their fuel. Similarly, athletes should not think of water as excess weight; rather, they should be concerned with minimizing excess fat weight.*

the body's *fat* weight.

"Ideal percent fat" can only be achieved by understanding the concept of caloric balance, because an understanding of this balance allows one to manipulate the body's fat weight. Two factors influence caloric balance: caloric input (the amount of food we eat) and caloric expenditure (the level of physical activity). If you consume or eat more Calories than your body requires, the balance will be "tipped." The extra Calories will be stored as fat in the adipose or fat cells, causing body composition to change. This increase in the stored fat means that the percent fat will go up. If the level of physical activity is also reduced, the muscles will become smaller and thus will not weigh as much as before. Therefore, a decreasing level of activity coupled with an increased caloric expenditure can result in a much faster rise in percent fat than would occur if just too many Calories were being consumed. Furthermore, the body weight will be affected differently by these two sets of circumstances. If you increase your caloric consumption and maintain the same amount of physical activity, your body weight will go up as you gain fat pounds. But if caloric consumption

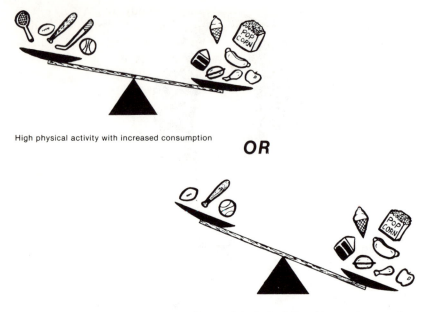

High physical activity with increased consumption

OR

Decreased physical activity and increased consumption

Figure 7.3. *Body fat is increased by increasing the caloric consumption. An even faster increase in body fat will occur if increased caloric consumption is accompanied by decreased activity.*

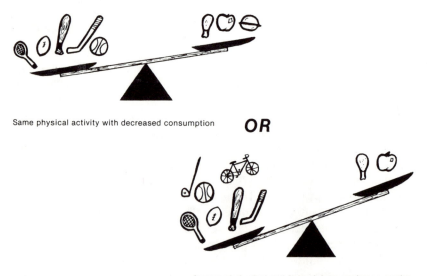

Same physical activity with decreased consumption

OR

Increased physical activity and decreased consumption

Figure 7.4. *Fat loss will occur if the caloric consumption is lower than caloric expenditure, and an even more rapid fat loss will occur if caloric restriction is accompanied by increased caloric expenditure.*

increases and physical activity decreases, the body weight may not increase a great deal because fat gains are offset by losses of lean or muscle tissue. In other words, the increases in body weight due to stored fat will be partially offset by the losses in lean or muscle tissue due to the decrease in physical activity. So while the balance may be "tipped," the body weight does not actually tell you how "damaging" the caloric imbalance is because the weight shown on your scale does not measure body composition.

Also, decreasing caloric intake may tip the balance in the opposite direction. Again, the effect of this procedure on body fat may be misleading if consideration is not given to the level of physical activity as well as the amount of decrease in caloric consumption. For example, if the numbers of Calories being consumed is decreased and the physical activity level is not very high, the body weight will drop, but the drop will be from lost lean tissue or muscle tissue as well as fat. Under these circumstances, the decrease in the number of Calories eaten is not sufficient to cover the caloric costs of the athlete's day-to-day activities. The body, however, has a backup mechanism—a safety device for just such occasions. The low number of Calories being consumed causes the blood sugar level to drop, and this triggers the release of several hormones. As discussed in chapter 4, these hormones are very important in that they allow the muscles to burn their stored glycogen and fat. They also allow liver to release its stored glucose so that the nerves have a fuel supply. In addition, some of

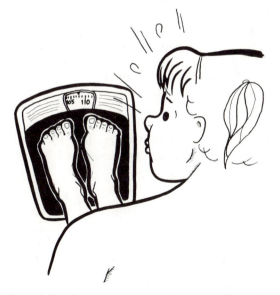

Figure 7.5. *Scale weights do not evaluate body composition; they do not tell athletes or their coaches the full story.*

these hormones (the glucocorticoids) cause the proteins in the muscle or lean tissue to be broken down. The amino acids from these muscle proteins are then taken in the blood to the liver, where the liver converts them into sugar. Thus, even after the liver's initial glycogen stores are depleted, the liver can continue to supply glucose to the blood so that nerve cells have adequate fuel. This process of breaking down protein is so effective that the liver can actually make more glucose than can be used by the nerve tissue. Consequently, the "extra" glucose is converted to fat and stored.

Surprising as it may seem, dieting, especially crash dieting, can actually *increase* the fat content. Although the body weight will decrease under these conditions, the percent fat will increase. Such a situation would certainly not enhance an athlete's physical efficiency. Therefore, we have provided a series of nutritional guidelines for losing fat weight.

Nutritional Guidelines for Fat Loss

Guideline 1: Weight loss should come from the fat stores in the body.

Losing only fat weight will help to ensure physical efficiency. The amount of fat weight that needs to be lost must be determined by evaluating the body's fat content, as described in chapter 2. By following those procedures you can tell athletes exactly how many pounds of fat they need to lose. For example, if you used the caliper technique and found that Elmo, a high school cross country runner, has a current percent fat of 13.0%, you would know that his current percent fat is higher than the ideal of 7% fat. Then, by doing the calculation on the recording form discussed in chapter 2, (see Table 7.1) you would be able to tell Elmo that he needs to lose 9 lbs of fat to reduce his percent fat to 7%.

Guideline No.2: Body fat should be reduced by using both reduced caloric consumption (dieting) and increased caloric expenditure (physical activity).

This guideline is important in that it will help to ensure that the weight loss is from the body's fat stores and *not* from the lean tissue. Remember, fat reduction is the goal!

Guideline No. 3: Reduce body fat gradually.

The caloric balance should be adjusted so fat losses never exceed 4 lbs a week. A weekly fat loss of 1-2 lbs is actually more desirable because the body's protective mechanism will cause lean tissue losses

Table 7.1

Elmo's Ideal Weight

Name _____Elmo_____ Age __14_____

Date _____ Weight __135_____lbs

Ideal Weight Prediction __126__ lbs   Weight to Lose/Gain ____9__ lbs

Skinfolds

	#1	#2	#3	Average
Triceps	5 mm	4 mm	5 mm	4.75 mm
Subscapular	10.5 mm	10 mm	10 mm	10 mm

Predicted % fat as read from the appropriate skinfold table = __13_ %

Body Wt. × Fat = Fat Weight   Body Weight − Fat Weight = LBW

135 lbs × .13 = 17.55 lbs   135 lbs − 17.55 lbs = 117 lbs

$$\text{Ideal Body Weight} = \frac{\text{LBW}}{(100\% - \text{Ideal \% Fat})}$$

$$\frac{117}{(100\% - 7\%)} = \underline{\qquad} \text{lbs}$$

$$\frac{117}{.93} = \underline{126} \text{ lbs}$$

---

if weight is lost at a faster rate. Also, a slower rate of weight loss produces less mental strain. Because each pound of fat is equivalent to about 3,500 kcal, the extent to which the caloric balance scales must be "tipped" to achieve the desired fat loss can be calculated by multiplying the number of pounds of desired fat loss by 3,500. Elmo needed to lose 9 lbs of fat; thus by multiplying 3,500 by 9, it can be determined that he needs to tip his caloric balance scales by 31,500 kcal. Because half of these Calories should be accounted for through dieting and half through increased physical activity, Elmo needs to restrict his diet by 15,700 kcal and increase his activity by 15,750 kcal. The time in which it will take Elmo to accomplish his task can now be determined. If you want Elmo to lose a pound per week, just divide 3,500 into the total number of kcal. If you want him to lose 2 lbs a week, divide by 7,000 kcal; for 3 lbs per week divide by 10,500 kcal; and if you want him to lose 4 lbs per week, divide by 14,000 kcal.

If Elmo has 5 weeks until his first race and you have decided that he should lose 2 lbs per week, Elmo must increase his caloric expenditure by 3,500 Calories a week or 500 Calories a day. In addition, Elmo must decrease his caloric intake by 3,500 Calories a week or 500 Calories a day. But before he can reduce his caloric consumption, he needs to know his approximate caloric requirement or need. This brings us to the fourth nutritional guideline.

Guideline 4: Caloric requirements should be assessed on the basis of age, body surface area, growth, and physical activity levels.

There is no single specific requirement for everyone; each of us has different nutritional needs. The reason for this variability in caloric need is related to how we use the Calories in the food that we eat. Basically, we use food: (a) to provide the energy to perform the automatic functions that sustain life (heart function, breathing, digestion, etc.), (b) to provide the energy for moving body parts as during

Table 7.2

Calorie Levels for Children

	Age	Number of Calories (Kcal)
Boys	1-3	1,300
and	3-6	1,600
Girls	6-9	2,100
	9-12	2,400
Boys	12-15	3,000
	15-18	3,400
	9-12	2,200
Girls	12-15	2,500
	15-18	2,300

Table 7.3

**Caloric Costs of Daily Activities
for Individuals of Varying Weights**[a]

	Calories/Min		
Activity	110 lb	150 lb	190 lb
Billiards	2.1	2.9	3.6
Carpentry	2.6	3.5	4.5
Circuit training	9.3	12.6	15.9
Cooking (males)	2.4	3.3	4.1
Cooking (females)	2.9	3.1	3.9
Eating (sitting)	1.2	1.6	2.0
Sitting quietly	1.1	1.4	1.8
Running (9 min/mile)	9.7	13.1	16.6
Running (6 min/mile)	13.9	17.3	20.8

[a]For a more complete list, see Appendix G.

physical activity, (c) to provide the energy and *nutrients* for the growth and repair of tissues. As a general guideline, the Food and Nutrition Board recommends the Calorie levels for children presented in Table 7.2.

The values in this table, however, do not take individual variability and more importantly physical training into consideration; the youngster who participates in several hours of vigorous activity will require more Calories than a sedentary classmate. In addition, the type of activity makes a difference. As shown in Table 7.3, the caloric cost of activities varies greatly. Another factor which influences the caloric cost of an activity is weight. Most energy cost charts have been based on the energy costs of a 150-lb adult. A person who weighs only 110 lbs will burn considerably fewer Calories for a given activity than a person who weighs 150 lbs. Consequently, the charts which depict caloric cost values in kcal per pound of body weight per minute are the most accurate type.

In spite of all these problems with predicting one's caloric requirement, some very accurate techniques for determining the caloric requirements of athletes are available. These will be discussed later in this chapter.

Up to this point, the focus of attention has centered on the energy value of food. Although food does indeed provide energy for our bodies, this is not its only value. It also has nutrient value.

Guideline No. 5: The daily caloric requirement of a young athlete should be obtained from a balanced diet.

A balanced diet will ensure that the nutrient needs as well as the caloric needs of the body are met. For instance, it is possible to eat the necessary number of Calories by consuming only cakes and cookies. Such a diet, however, would not supply all of the essential amino acids (proteins), the appropriate vitamins and minerals, or the essential fatty acids. Shown in Table 7.4 is the comparison between the nutrients in cupcakes made with a mix, eggs, milk, and chocolate icing with the nutrients in eggs alone and skim milk alone. Most of the protein, iron, potassium, and Vitamin A in the cupcakes come from the eggs, and the thiamine and riboflavin come from the eggs and milk. If you ate the same amount of egg instead of cupcakes, you would consume less than half the Calories and over twice the nutrient value!

Having your athletes eat selections from the four basic food groups will ensure that they eat a balanced diet. The four basic groups and their recommended portions are listed in Table 7.5.

Guideline 6: Make daily water consumption an absolute must!

As we have repeatedly emphasized, weight loss should come from the fat stores, the body's true "excess weight," and not the body's vital water supply. *Never* go without water.

Now that you know the six guidelines for losing fat weight, you are ready to learn how to implement a fat loss program. The steps for doing this are presented next.

Weight Loss Steps

Step 1: Determine the body composition 6-8 weeks prior to the season and predict the ideal body weight.

By completing the procedures described in chapter 2, you can show your athletes how much of their body mass is comprised of fat and can give them individualized fat loss goals. Remember, you must not let your athletes get carried away and try to reach 0% fat. In doing so, they will not only jeopardize their athletic careers but also their physical health. All human beings need some body fat!

Step 2: Set up a weight loss timetable.

Once the body composition has been evaluated, the hardest part is yet to come. That is, the athlete must get down to and maintain this "ideal weight" all season. Do not be in a hurry to have your athletes reach their optimal weight and do not use the word diet. Instead, en-

Table 7.4

Comparison of Nutrient Value of Cupcakes, Eggs, and Skim Milk

One pound of:	Food Energy Calories	Protein Grams	Carbohydrate Grams	Calcium Milligrams	Phosphorus Milligrams	Iron Milligrams	Sodium Milligrams	Potassium Milligrams	Vitamin A International Units	Thiamine Milligrams	Riboflavin Milligrams	Niacin Milligrams	Ascorbic Acid Milligrams
Cupcake mix made with eggs, milk, and chocolate icing	1,624	20.4	268.5	590	894	3.6	1,520	531	770	.16	.49	1.0	trace
Eggs	739	58.5	4.1	245	930	10.4	553	585	5,350	.48	1.35	.3	0
Skim milk	163	16.3	23.1	549	431	.2	236	658	20	.16	.80	.3	5

Table 7.5

The Four Basic Food Groups

Food Group	Servings Per Day
MILK 1 c milk, yogurt, or calcium equivalent (1½ oz or 45 gm cheddar cheese; 1 c pudding; 1¾ c ice cream; 2 c cottage cheese)	3 for child 4 for adolescent 2 for adult
MEAT 2 oz cooked, lean meat, fish, poultry, or protein equivalent (2 eggs; 2 oz or 60 gm cheddar cheese; ½ c cottage cheese; 1 c dried beans or peas; 4 tbsp peanut butter; 2 oz nuts)	2 3-4 for athletes in heavy strength training program
FRUIT-VEGETABLE[a] ½ c cooked or juice 1 c raw	4, including 1 from the vitamin C group, 1 from vitamin A group
GRAIN[a] Whole-grain bread; 1 tortilla; 1 c whole-grain cereal; ½ c cooked cereal, rice, pasta, grits	4

[a]If additional Calories are necessary for additional energy, increase the number of fruit and vegetable servings.

courage athletes to view the weight control process as a valuable part of life in general, not just as a short-term diet.

The weight-loss timetable is a valuable tool for achieving optimal weight. Selma, for instance, is a 157-lb female high school basketball player whose optimal weight is 145; thus, she must lose 12 lbs. Because evaluation of body composition should be completed at least 6 weeks prior to the basketball season, she should have at least 6 weeks to achieve her desired weight. Weekly goals for the fat loss project like those shown in Table 7.6 can guide her. Notice that in the table a line has been drawn from the point at which her current weight and the

Table 7.6

Weight Loss Timetable

Name _Selma_   Dates: _Oct. 17, 1981_ to _Dec. 1, 1981_
Goal _145 lbs_

Starting Weight (lbs)

157 · 156 · 155 · 154 · 153 · 152 · 151 · 150 · 149 · 148 · 147 · 146 · 145

1st 2nd 3rd 4th 5th 6th

Weeks

beginning of the first week intersect to the point at which her optimal weight and the end of the sixth week intersect. This line is a "goal line" and shows that Selma must have a weekly goal of 2 lbs of fat loss in order to lose 12 lbs in 6 weeks.

Two times a week, on the same days and at about the same time, Selma should weigh herself and record the weight on the weight loss chart. If her weight plot points are below the goal line, it is an indication that she is losing weight too rapidly. This means that she is losing lean or muscle tissues as well as fat stores, and she must therefore be

Table 7.7

Caloric Intake Chart

Eating Time	Food Eaten	Amount	Caloric Value (Kcal)
Breakfast			
Snack			
Lunch			
Snack			
Dinner			

discouraged from becoming overzealous about losing weight. If, on the other hand, Selma's weight plot points are above the goal line, her fat reduction is not on schedule. This means that she needs to reevaluate her eating habits as well as her exercise program.

Step 3: Record food consumption and energy expenditures for three typical days.

This step may seem like it requires a lot of time, but ultimately it will be time well spent. Use charts similar to those shown in Tables 7.7 and 7.8 at least 1 week before beginning the weight loss program. This will allow you to accurately determine the normal caloric intake and normal caloric expenditure values for each athlete. Also, the records will allow you to help athletes see if they are fulfilling their body's nutrient as well as caloric needs.

The caloric intake chart shown in Table 7.7 is merely a listing of all

Table 7.8

Caloric Expenditure Chart

Activity	Duration	Total Calories Burned (Kcal)

the foods and liquids your athletes consume. The caloric values for many foods may be found in Appendix D. The older the athlete, the more complex the chart can be and the less you as a coach will have to be involved in the recording and Calorie-counting processes. Table 7.8, a caloric expenditure chart, helps athletes to keep track of all activities they complete each day. Consequently, the hours in the duration column should add up to 24.

As was explained before, if one is not gaining or losing weight and one's physical activity lifestyle is not changing, there is a perfect or near perfect balance between caloric intake and caloric expenditure. Thus, by using the caloric intake chart you can determine the caloric needs of individual athletes.

This individual value is important because it allows you to help athletes establish individualized caloric intake and output goals. By knowing the caloric requirement, you will not have to use caloric requirement charts to predict the caloric needs of specific athletes. Instead, by record-keeping, you and your athletes will account for individual differences in body chemistry, skeletal height, amount of initial body fat, and other subtle factors which make each athlete unique. These individual differences necessitate the use of individual caloric restriction levels. Once the caloric intake charts and the caloric expenditure charts have been completed for a typical week, this individualization can begin.

For example, according to her charts, Selma consumes an average of 3,100 Calories per day and normally burns the same amount, and she must achieve a fat loss of 2 lbs or 7,000 Calories per week. Because half of these Calories should come from increased physical activity

Table 7.9

Selma's Caloric Restriction and Caloric Expenditure Chart

Day	New kcal Intake	Less Than Normal	New kcal Expenditure	More Than Normal
1	2,600[a]	− 500	3,600[a]	+ 500
2	2,600	− 500	3,600	+ 500
3	2,600	− 500	3,600	+ 500
4	2,600	− 500	3,600	+ 500
5	2,600	− 500	3,600	+ 500
6	2,600	− 500	3,600	+ 500
7	2,600	− 500	3,600	+ 500
Total 7		3,500 fewer kcal eaten /week		3,500 extra kcal being burned /week

[a]Before the weight loss program, Selma's normal caloric intake was 3,100 kcal and her normal expenditure was 3,100 kcal.

and half from caloric restriction, Selma needs to cut out 3,500 Calories a week or 500 Calories a day (3,500 ÷ 7days = 500). Likewise, she needs to increase her physical activities so she expends an additional 3,500 Calories a week or 500 a day. (Appendix G provides some information for determining the caloric cost of exercise. For example, because running 1 mile uses about 100 Calories for someone Selma's size, Selma would have to run a total of 5 miles per day to expend the 500 extra Calories.)

Step 4: Never allow caloric intake to go below 1,800-2,000 kcal/day.

This fourth step involves the decisions for actually accounting for the caloric equivalents that will bring about the fat reduction. Table 7.9 shows Selma's new caloric restriction and expenditure levels. These levels, remember, are based on her individual needs.

In other words, the normal caloric consumption value of 3,100 Calories was used to determine how many Calories she will be able to consume on a daily basis during her fat loss program. Also, by knowing that she should be consuming only 2,600 kcal, Selma can

Table 7.10

**Suggested Maximum Rates of Weight Loss
for Athletes of Varying Size**

	Total Body Weight		
Before Season	98-125 lbs	126-165 lbs	166 lbs and up
Per week restrictions	Eat 250 kcals less per day × 7 days = 1,750 kcal	Eat 500 kcals less per day × 7 days = 3,500 kcal	Eat 750 kcals less per day × 7 days = 5,250 kcal
Weight loss due to caloric restriction	½ lb/wk	1 lb/wk	1½ lbs/wk
Weight loss due to increased expenditure	½ lb/wk	1 lb/wk	1½ lb/wk
Total weight loss	1 lb/wk	2 lbs/wk	3 lbs/wk

periodically evaluate her food intake by using the daily recording chart.

Obviously, not all athletes will have a 2 lb per week goal. For instance, a 184-lb athlete can probably afford to cut out a few more calories than can a 105-lb athlete. Table 7.10 should help you and your athletes to decide upon some realistic goals.

A concept underlying Table 7.10 is that an active athlete should never go below a 2,000 Calorie intake per day; smaller male and female athletes should not go below 1,800 Calories. To adhere to this stipulation, the smaller athletes will not be able to restrict their caloric intake as severely as will the larger athlete and will have to rely more heavily upon caloric expenditure. By adhering to this caloric consumption minimum, the athlete will help ensure that the nutrient needs of training and *growth* are met. (Occasionally a doctor will prescribe a diet of less than 1,800-2,000 Calories, but in such cases,

Table 7.11

Wrestler's Diet for Losing Weight

Want to lose weight? Try this. You are guaranteed to lose weight (or your health).

Monday	Breakfast	Weak tea
	Lunch	1 bouillon cube in ¼ cup of diluted water
	Dinner	1 pigeon thigh
		3 oz prune juice (gargle only)

Tuesday	Breakfast	Scraped crumbs from burned toast
	Lunch	1 doughnut hole (without sugar)
		1 glass of dehydrated water
	Dinner	2 grains of corn meal (broiled)

Wednesday	Breakfast	Boiled out stains of table cloth
	Lunch	½ doz poppy seeds
	Dinner	Bee's knees and mosquitos' knuckles sauteed in vinegar

Thursday	Breakfast	Shredded eggshell skins
	Lunch	1 belly button from a navel orange
	Dinner	3 eyes from Irish potato (diced)

Friday	Breakfast	2 lobster antennae
	Lunch	1 guppy fin
	Dinner	Fillet of soft shellcrab slaw

Saturday	Breakfast	4 chopped banana seeds
	Lunch	Broiled butterfly liver
	Dinner	Jellyfish vertebrae a la bookbinder

Sunday	Breakfast	Pickled hummingbird tongue
	Lunch	Prime ribs of tadpole
		Aroma of empty custard pie plate
	Dinner	Tossed paprika and (1) clover leaf salad

Note. All meals to be eaten under a microscope to avoid extra portions.

Table 7.12

A Sample 2,000 kcal Reducing Diet

BREAKFAST
½ cup grapefruit juice (50 kcal)
1 glass skim milk (90 kcal)
1 piece of buttered whole wheat
  toast (100 kcal)
1 small bowl of nonsugar-coated
  cereal (with milk) (100 kcal)

LUNCH
Tuna sandwich (270 kcal)
  Slice tomato and lettuce
  (50 kcal)
1 glass skim milk (90 kcal)
1 banana (100 kcal)

DINNER
½ glass skim milk (45 kcal)
Tossed salad with low calorie
  Italian dressing (150 kcal)
½ cup green beans (15 kcal)
1 medium baked potato
  (100 kcal)
4 oz baked chicken (215 kcal)
2 oatmeal with raisin cookies
  (120 kcal)

SNACKS
1 orange (80 kcal)
1 peanut butter (1 tablespoon)
  and jelly (1 teaspoon) sandwich (285 kcal)
½ glass skim milk (45 kcal)

---

vitamin and mineral supplements will also be prescribed.) Although the word diet often provokes the idea of an eating plan such as that shown in Table 7.11, the one in Table 7.12 is a much more realistic—and nutritional—plan.

Step 5: Athletes should eat foods from the four basic food groups.

Not only should the foods be from the four basic food groups, they should be low in caloric value and high in bulk. Foods of this nature include salads, bran flakes, fresh fruits, and raw vegetables. These are foods that "fill you up, not out."

Step 6: Encourage athletes not to skip meals and to spread out the calories consumed.

Reducing athletes may eat five times a day—three meals and two snacks. The "snacks," however, should be of high protein or fruit sugar in nature and not candy or junk food. Eating five times a day spreads out caloric intake over the day, keeping the appetite more satisfied. In addition, research has demonstrated that the gastrointestinal tract is less efficient if the food intake is spread out over five to six meals, meaning that fewer Calories are absorbed into the bloodstream. If only one meal is consumed, the gastrointestinal tract is very efficient in extracting all available Calories. It has also

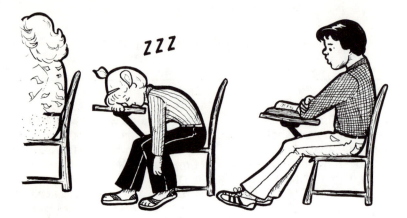

Figure 7.6. *Missing breakfast can make students sleepy and impair their schoolwork.*

been shown that a missed breakfast can reduce an individual's effectiveness by 25%, which can make it hard for young athletes to do their schoolwork.

Step 7: Drink one quart of water for every 1,000 kcal eaten.

Water is one of the important elements of the weight loss program and it has no caloric value. There is not one single Calorie in water. Therefore, athletes should cultivate good water-drinking habits. (Some modification of this guide will be discussed in chapter 10.)

Step 8: Utilize behavior modification techniques to help maintain motivation during the weight loss period.

Physiological factors are not the only factors which athletes losing fat weight need to consider; the psychological side of weight loss is also important. Thus, psychologists have suggested a number of "tricks" to help people trying to lose weight. Many of these tricks or modifications of them will be valuable to athletes.

For example, to help keep athletes motivated, a compilation of physical and psychological penalties charts might be advantageous. A physical penalties chart is a list of all the bad physical outcomes of using the "roller coaster approach" to making weight, whereas the psychological penalties chart consists of all the bad psychological feelings associated with this approach. Posting these charts in a conspicuous place can provide the incentive to continue a gradual fat loss program.

Motivation can also be enhanced by using incentives and rewards. Parents and coaches in particular can play an important role in this

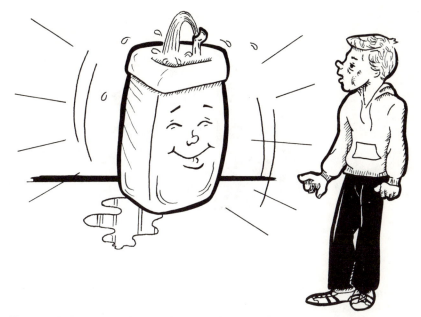

Figure 7.7. *Athletes and water fountains should become good friends.*

process. Using the weight loss chart as a record of achieved goals, parents and coaches can acknowledge the realization of each goal with many types of rewards, including:

1. Doing something special with the family or a friend (other than eating);

2. Treating the athlete to an extra hour of sleep Saturday morning;

3. Allowing the athlete to choose a favorite program on the family television set;

4. Going on a shopping trip for a needed or desired object (clothes, records, books, etc.); or

5. Excusing the athlete from a specific chore on a given day (washing dishes, taking out trash, etc.).

These are only a few of the ideas which psychologists have proposed. For additional ideas, you may wish to obtain some of the books on utilizing behavior modification to aid with weight loss (see Appendix H).

Step 9: Use judgment and objective criteria to determine if athletes are losing weight properly.

The following questions should help you implement this step.

1. Is the athlete maintaining muscular strength or is it deteriorating? (Periodically test strength.)

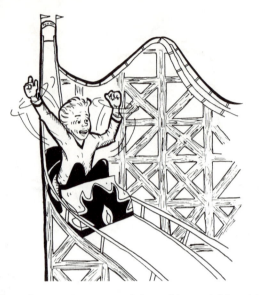

Figure 7.8. *The roller coaster approach to making weight must be avoided; instead, athletes should pursue long-term fat control programs.*

2. Is the athlete maintaining speed and quickness? (Again, actual measurements allow you to evaluate progress.)

3. Does the athlete appear to "wear down" at the end of practice games and matches?

4. Does the athlete appear lethargic and inattentive in classes, at practice, or at home?

5. Has the athlete demonstrated a marked change in personality or disposition during the weight loss period?

Step 10: Once athletes have reached their optimal weight, ensure that they maintain it.

You can help athletes by providing frequent weigh-ins so that their weight does not "bounce" up and down. If this is allowed to occur and athletes are forced to crash diet, they will be exposed to three physiological disadvantages. First, they will deplete the carbohydrate stores in their muscles from the 24-48 hours of semistarvation. These stores constitute the quick source of explosive energy athletes need. Second, the chemical and water balance in the blood and fluid around the cells will be upset. This also will detract from performance efficiency. Third, the roller coaster approach to making weight prevents the body from acclimatizing and stabilizing. Athletes' vitality will be lowered, weakness will set in, and athletes will become more susceptible to colds and infection.

As you can see, helping athletes to stay at or maintain their ideal

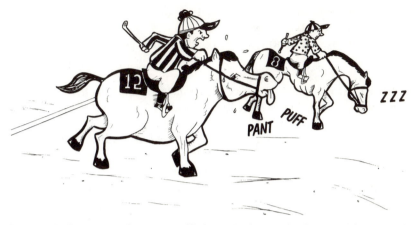

Figure 7.9. *Optimal performance efficiency is the result of optimal fat control. Few fat horses will cross the line first, but neither will scrawny, dehydrated horses be found in the winner's circle.*

weight throughout the season provides them with some nutritional conditioning. In fact, you are helping athletes to develop sound, life-long dietary habits.

Summary

In conclusion, we would like to present you with a simplified checklist of the steps to follow for sensible weight loss.

Step 1. Determine the body composition 6-8 weeks prior to season and predict the ideal body weight.

Step 2. Set up a weight loss timetable.

Step 3. Keep an accurate, 7-day record of food consumption and energy expended.

Step 4. Never allow caloric intake to go below 1,800-2,000 kcal per day. (Larger athletes may lose weight at a more rapid rate than smaller ones.)

Step 5. The foods eaten should be taken from the four basic food groups and should be low in caloric content and high in bulk.

Step 6. Encourage athletes to not skip meals and to spread out the Calories consumed. (Remember, snacks should be high in protein or fruit sugar; they should not be candy or junk food.)

Step 7. Ensure that athletes drink one quart of water for every 1,000 kcal eaten.

Step 8. Utilize behavior modification techniques to help maintain motivation during the weight loss period.

Step 9. Use good judgment and objective criteria in monitoring the weight loss period.

Step 10. Once the optimal weight is reached, make sure the athletes maintain it!

Chapter 8
How to Gain Weight

In chapter 7, we discussed how you can help your athletes lose excess fat weight to improve their physical efficiency. Not all sports, however, have the same performance demands, and thus, their characteristics of physical efficiency vary. Some athletes such as the shot putter, discus thrower, football lineman, and the heavyweight wrestler require maximal muscle mass, needing both bulk and explosive strength. Remember, however, these athletes should increase their muscle weight, not just their body weight. Additional fat weight will only be "excess baggage"; it will not contribute to athletes' explosive strength potential. Furthermore, excess fat predisposes athletes to a number of different diseases and other health problems.

Increases in the muscle mass or lean body weight are of considerable importance to performance success in some sports. Therefore, the guidelines for gaining lean weight presented in this chapter supplement the fat loss guidelines discussed in the last chapter.

Although gaining lean weight is considerably different than losing fat weight, the concept of

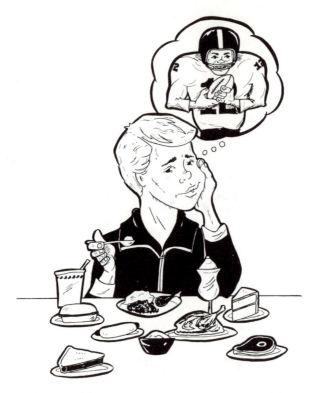

Figure 8.1. *Gaining lean weight takes more than dreams and desserts, it takes intense resistive exercise.*

caloric balance is the same. The emphasis, however, is on high rather than reduced caloric intake. Furthermore, high caloric intake without increases in body fat are only possible if they are balanced by intense resistive exercise. With this in mind let's look at the eight guidelines for gaining lean weight.

Guideline 1: Consider the medical history of the athlete.

No athlete should participate in a weight gaining program if his or her family has a medical history of heart disease or high blood pressure. Furthermore, whenever possible, a blood test should be given to determine if abnormal levels of lipids or fats are present in the blood plasma. Blood pressure can also be used to determine whether a weight gain program should be undertaken or continued. If the blood pressure is high initially, a weight gain program should not be started, or if the blood pressure increases during the course of the program, the program should be terminated.

Guideline 2: Increase caloric consumption by 2,500 Calories for each

pound of lean tissue to be gained.

One pound of lean tissue is equivalent to about 2,500 Calories (kcal) of potential energy. Fat, remember, contains about 3,500 kcal per pound. The difference in the number of Calories between these two tissues reflects the composition of the tissues. Lean tissues, such as muscle and nerve tissue, contain more protein, carbohydrate, and water than does fat tissue.

Guideline 3: Increased caloric consumption should be coupled with heavy resistive exercise to gain lean weight or muscle weight.

In chapter 7, you learned that if the caloric intake exceeds the daily caloric output, the excess Calories are stored as fat. However, if athletes not only increase their caloric intake but also work with weights and other resistive devices, their body will use the extra Calories to build muscle tissue and other lean tissues.

By resistive exercise, we mean strength development exercises. (We'll discuss these exercises in more detail in chapter 9.) Although weight training programs of this type will result in muscle growth, they can also be very stressful on growing bones. Therefore, these types of heavy strength-training programs should not begin until after puberty when the growth of the long bones is nearing completion. Prior to this time, athletes can still use weight training, but with higher numbers of repetitions and lighter weights.

Guideline 4: Weight gain should be slow and gradual.

Caloric intake should not exceed caloric output by more than 1,000 to 1,500 kcal per day. In other words, there is a limit as to how fast lean weight gain can be accomplished. If too many Calories are consumed too fast, some of the weight gained will be fat weight.

In addition to limiting the caloric intake to 1,000-1,500 kcal over caloric output, the increased Calorie consumption should also be limited to those days on which resistive training is done. Because it takes at least 48 hours for the muscles to recover, heavy weight work should not be undertaken more frequently than every other day; consequently, increased caloric consumption should also be limited to every other day.

For example, let us say that Duke, an 18-year-old interior lineman, would like to gain 10 lbs of lean tissue, which is equivalent to 25,000 Calories. He works out with weights 3 days a week, so if he increases his caloric consumption by 1,000 kcal a day for each of those 3 workout days, he will eat 3,000 extra Calories each week. This means that he will need a little over 8 weeks to gain the desired lean weight. Just as losing fat weight takes time, so too does gaining lean tissue. Do not allow your athletes to become impatient; excessive Calories will only be stored as fat.

Guideline 5: Avoid extremely large meals.

Increased caloric consumption is better achieved by adding snacks or meals rather than eating one or two very large meals (see Table 8.1). More total Calories can be consumed by following this eating pattern. Also, spreading out the caloric consumption throughout the day builds better lifetime dietary habits. When the athlete no longer needs to gain weight, the caloric intake can be reduced by cutting out snacks, still leaving three meals a day.

Guideline 6: Consume the largest portion of the caloric intake early in the day.

First, this helps to ensure that all requisite amino acids and other food components are eaten in close proximity, making it more likely that these substances will all be available to the body for tissue formation. Some recent research has shown that all of the constituents for building new tissues must be available simultaneously. The body does not seem to be able to hold what is eaten for breakfast until the rest of the "ingredients" are eaten for lunch. This is a major reason for eating balanced meals.

The second reason for eating a larger portion of the caloric intake early in the day is that this food can serve as the fuel for the active part of the day. A large meal eaten in the evening has a greater tendency to result in fat deposits than does a substantial breakfast. This is true not only for athletes but for everyone.

Guideline 7: Avoid excessive amounts of animal fats and salty foods.

Research has demonstrated that a diet high in saturated fats (animal fats) may lead to an increased incidence of cardiovascular disease. In addition, the high salt content of the typical American diet is thought to play a role in causing hypertension. Although animal fats should be minimized, vegetable oils (except coconut oil) are an important part of the high Calorie diet because fats are a high density food. A high density food is one which contains a large number of Calories for a given volume. Not all high density foods are good for a sensible weight-gain program, however.

For example, Jay, a basketball player needing to gain weight, heard that pop is high in Calories. So he decided to gain weight by drinking extra pop. Each evening after practice he managed to pour 12 to 14 cans of pop down his throat, representing between 1,600 and 1,960 kcal. Although Jay consumed a substantial number of Calories, he

Table 8.1

A Sample High Calorie Diet for Gaining Muscle Weight (6,027 kcal)

BREAKFAST
1 glass skim milk (90 kcal)
1 glass cranberry juice cocktail (165 kcal)
1 soft-boiled egg (80 kcal)
2 pieces of whole wheat toast (130 kcal)
1½ teaspoons margarine (105 kcal)
1 tablespoon jelly (50 kcal)
½ cup granola (260 kcal)

LUNCH
1 glass skim milk (90 kcal)
1 chicken breast—6 oz (310 kcal)
1 cup rice with cheese sauce (315 kcal)
Tossed salad with dressing (200 kcal)
1 cup fruit cocktail (190 kcal)
4 oatmeal and raisin cookies (240 kcal)

DINNER
Large baked potato with sour cream and margarine (280 kcal)
6 oz of baked fish (300 kcal)
1 cup creamed broccoli casserole with sesame seeds on top (350 kcal)
½ cup of cottage cheese with pears (200 kcal)
2 dinner rolls with margarine (310 kcal)
1 piece of apple pie (400 kcal)

SNACKS
1 cup dried peaches and other dried fruits (420 kcal)
1 pt of sherbet (400 kcal)
1 glass of orange juice (80 kcal)
½ cup peanuts (392 kcal)
1 milkshake (320 kcal)
½ cup gorp [granola, dried fruits, chocolate bits, nuts, and coconut (250 kcal)]
1 banana (100 kcal)

---

also destroyed his appetite for the evening. Consequently, he was not able to increase his total daily caloric consumption. Furthermore, drinking so much pop prevented him from getting a balance of nutrients. Finally, he was not building sound, lifetime eating habits. Jay's attempt to increase his caloric consumption would have been much more successful had he elected to eat foods that are high in Calories and low in bulk, such as those listed in Table 8.1.

Guideline 8: Do not use androgenic hormones or anabolic steroids to promote weight gain.

Research shows that taking the male sex hormone, testosterone, and synthetic hormones such as Dianabol® in concert with weight training programs and high caloric diets will bring about an increase in muscle tissue. But there is no agreement as to whether this increase will improve muscular strength and endurance. More importantly, anyone who takes anabolic steroids before he or she stops growing is likely to stunt growth because these steroids can prematurely arrest the growth zones at the end of the long bones. Other side effects of these substances are acne, excessive body hair, and enlargement of the breasts (because some of the hormones are converted to the female hormone, estrogen). Due to these factors, as well as the ethical considerations, the use of anabolic steroids has no place in the weight gain program of athletes—young or old! (For a more complete review of the problem, the excellent position paper of the American College of Sports Medicine has been included in Appendix I of this book.)

Now that you know the guidelines, let's take a look at the steps for implementing a weight gain program.

Step 1: Determine the optimal weight (6-8 weeks) prior to the season and decide upon the needed gain in muscle tissue.

Prior to the beginning of the sport season, the ideal playing weight of the athlete should be determined using the procedures presented in chapter 2. Use good, common sense when deciding if any athlete needs to gain weight. For example, if a football player has a lower body weight but a percent fat similar to his or her teammates and opponents, the need to gain lean tissue is apparent.

Step 2: Evaluate the potential effect of weight gain on the athlete's overall health.

As mentioned in Guideline 1, athletes who have high blood pressure or high blood lipids should not be encouraged to gain weight.

Step 3: Determine the athlete's caloric intake and output.

A week's record of the individual's caloric consumption and caloric expenditure should be recorded using forms similar to those shown in Table 7.7 and Table 7.8. Body weight, girth measurements, skinfold measurements, sprint times, and strength scores also should be recorded (see Table 8.2). These values can be used to evaluate the quality of the weight gain. For example, if weight goes up but waist girth and skinfolds do too, then it is likely that the weight gain is fat tissue. Similarly, if there are no increases in strength and the individual's sprint times and agility run times increase, the weight gain is obviously not enhancing the athlete's performance potential. Muscle girth measurements can also serve as objective criteria.

Step 4: Plot the weight gain goals on the weight gain timetable.

The caloric consumption and caloric expenditure information collected in Step 3 can be used to establish the weight gain timetable by

Table 8.2

Criteria for Evaluating Weight Gain

Purpose of the weight gain program _____

_____

Weight gain goal _____ Target time _____

Criteria	Date	Date	Date	Date	Date	Date
1. Body weight 2. Subscapular skinfold 3. Triceps skinfold 4. 20 yd sprint time 5. 50 yd sprint time 6. Waist girth 7. Upper-arm girth 8. Calf girth 9. Chest girth 10. Bench press 11. Other						

plotting a "weight gain goal line," as shown in Table 8.3. For example, let's say that you find Buddy needs to gain 10 lbs of lean tissue. You confer with him and decide to increase his food consumption by 1,000 calories on 3 training days per week. He should gain about 1 lb (1.2 to be exact) per week for a total of 8.3 weeks. To plot the goal line, place a dot at the intersection of the starting weight and the zero week line and another at the intersection of the desired weight and the final week; then draw a line connecting the two points. Sound familiar? It should; we used the same procedure in the previous chapter on losing weight. Buddy should weigh in twice a week, on the same days and at about the same time; then you or he should record those weights on the timetable. Buddy should also keep a record of his strength gains in conjunction with the weight training program. The evaluation of his skinfolds, sprint times, and agility should be kept weekly (see Table 8.2).

Table 8.3

Weight Gain Timetable

Name _Buddy_ _____ Dates: _July 6, 1981_ to _Aug. 24, 1981_

Goal: _Gain 10 lbs_ _____

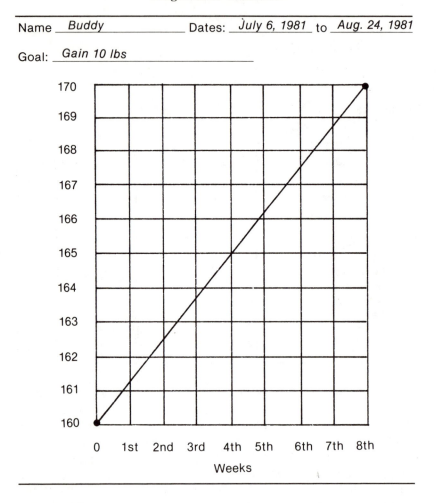

Step 5: Emphasize the consumption of high Calorie but nutritious snacks and meals.

When losing weight, emphasis is placed on high bulk foods such as cereals, grains, and salads. These types of food, however, are too filling to constitute a very high percentage of the weight gain dietary intake. Rather, high Calorie density foods must be eaten. Fats are just such a food, but care must be taken to avoid excessive amounts of animal fats. In addition, for energy management purposes, the athlete should be encouraged to indulge in low bulk carbohydrates which will provide the fuel for intense physical activity. It is *not* necessary that

Table 8.4

High Calorie Density Snacks

Nuts:
  Cashews
  Peanuts
  Almonds
  Walnuts
Coconuts
Milk
Chocolate milk
Sherbet (has the sugar calories without the animal fat of ice cream)
Sherbet sundaes with nuts, wheat germ, and coconut topping
Shakes and malts
Cheese
Dried fruit (without its water content, fruit is very high in Calories)
Peanut butter sandwiches

---

athletes gorge themselves with large quantities of expensive meat in order to "bulk" up on protein. Athletes need no more than 2 grams of protein per kilogram of body weight (1 gram per pound). Eating large quantities of red meat means eating not only protein but also large quantities of animal fat, and as you learned in chapter 7, neither of these are desirable in excess. Consequently, you need to discuss nutritious, high Calorie meal plans, such as those listed in Table 8.1, with your athletes and their parents. You should also introduce athletes to nutritious, high Calorie snacks like those shown in Table 8.4.

Step 6: Periodically evaluate the dietary intake.

Although athletes don't need to keep the caloric consumption and caloric expenditure charts on a daily basis, they should be continually aware of what types of foods to avoid, the number of Calories to consume, the type of Calories to consume, and the number of meals to eat. Remember, the purpose of these guidelines is not only to gain weight but also to promote positive lifetime dietary habits!

A particularly good habit to begin with is regulating protein consumption. Athletes are very interested in ensuring that their diets contain adequate protein, but they usually overestimate their protein needs and tend to select protein sources that are high in salt and animal fat. Consequently, your athletes and their parents should evaluate the quantity of protein consumed during a given day. This

Table 8.5

Protein Content of Typical Foods

Food	Grams of Protein per oz of Food
Eggs	6
Whole milk	18
Cottage cheese	4
Yogurt	1
Cheddar cheese	3
Tuna fish	8
Chicken	8
Steak	8
Hamburger	7
Liver	8
Pork Chops	5
Ham	5
Brewer's yeast	12
Wheat germ	8
Cotton seed flour	7.5
Soybean flour	7.5
Nuts	3-5

can be done by having the athlete use his or her caloric consumption charts and a chart similar to that found in Table 8.6. The amount of protein eaten can be approximated by using the information given in Table 8.5 or Appendix D. In addition, the information in Table 8.7 illustrates how emphasis upon the consumption of chicken, fish, and plant fats can significantly improve the quality of the weight gain diet.

Step 7: Use a weight training program to maintain lean tissue.

When the desired weight gain has been achieved, the excessive caloric consumption should be stopped and a maintenance weight training program begun. In addition, if the caloric expenditure is reduced when the season ends or an injury is incurred, the caloric intake should also be reduced. High caloric intake without increases in body fat are only possible if they are balanced by intensive resistive exercise.

Table 8.6

Evaluation of Athlete's Protein Consumption

Protein Source	Amount of Protein	High in Animal Fat
Two eggs	30 grams	Yes
Bacon (4 oz)	20 grams	Yes
Two hamburgers	42 grams	Yes
Steak dinner	128 grams	Yes
Four glasses of whole milk	100 grams	Yes
½ cup cottage cheese	32 grams	Yes
	352 grams	

Athlete's weight = 80 kg or 168 lbs
Athlete's protein need* = 120-160 grams/day

*(Wt. × 1.5 − 2.0 grams/kg = Protein need)
(80 kg × 1.5 grams/kg = 120 grams)
(80 kg × 2.0 grams/kg = 160 grams)

Protein consumed = 352 grams/day (This is more than needed.)

Summary

As in chapter 7, we have provided you with a simplified checklist of the steps to follow in helping your athletes gain muscle mass.

Step 1. Determine the optimal weight (6-8 weeks) prior to the season and decide upon the needed gain in muscle tissue.

Step 2. Arrange a physical examination for these athletes and, with the aid of a physician, determine if weight gain will be detrimental to the future health of the athlete.

Step 3. Gather information about the daily caloric consumption, daily caloric expenditure, initial body weight and body composition, initial muscular strength, initial muscle girth measurements, initial sprint speeds, and initial agility.

Step 4. Set up a weight gain timetable. (Remember that caloric in-

Table 8.7

Evaluation of Athlete's Protein Consumption

Protein Source	Amount of Protein	High in Animal Fat
Two glasses of 2% milk	50 grams	Some
Tuna fish sandwich	30 grams	No
Chicken (light meat)	90 grams	No
	170 grams	

Athlete's weight = 80 kg or 168 lbs
Athlete's protein need* = 120-180 grams/day

*(Wt. × 1.5 − 2.0 grams/kg = Protein need)
(80 kg × 1.5 grams/kg = 120 grams)

Protein consumed = 170 grams (This is about what is needed.)

take should not exceed caloric expenditure by more than 1,000-1,500 Calories.)

Step 5. Emhasize the consumption of high Calorie, but nutritious snacks and meals.

Step 6. Periodically evaluate the dietary intake to help foster a safe weight gain program and establish sound lifetime dietary habits.

Step 7. Once the athletes have reached their desired weight, reinforce maintenance strategies to help the athletes prevent weight gain from becoming accumulating fat pounds.

Chapter 9
Strength Training

Strength training is an important adjunct of weight control and energy management programs. Not only has "Mean" Joe Green of the Pittsburgh Steelers benefited from strength training, but so has Bill Rodgers, the winner of three consecutive Boston Marathons, as has gymnast Nadia Comaneci, Olympic gold medalist.

Strength development is important for athletes in almost all sports. Stronger muscles not only enable athletes to run faster, throw farther, jump higher, and move more efficiently, they also help prevent injuries by enhancing joint stability and facilitating body mobility. In addition to muscular strength, for some sports a large muscle mass is also important. For example, football linemen, weight event competitors, and wrestlers in the heavier weight class can use this mass to overcome inertia and generate momentum. Unfortunately, many athletes and their coaches have overemphasized the need for mass. As a result, the "bigger is better myth" has flourished, producing athletes who drag around pounds of excess fat weight.

Therefore, not only do you need to know how

to use the skinfold caliper and the guidelines for caloric balance, you also need to be aware of the basic principles of resistive exercise training so you can design strength development programs to help your athletes complete their weight control program.

The Principles of Resistive Exercise

The development of a good strength training program is really not that difficult, although we hear about many different approaches. There are three major training principles:

- The Gradual Overload Principle
- The SAID Principle
- The Principle of Reversibility

The Gradual Overload Principle

Strength training must be progressive; that is, the muscles must be required to do more and more work during successive workouts. Muscular strength is the ability of the nervous system to recruit or call into maximal operation the fibers of a muscle. Thus strength training is really the process of teaching the nervous system how to maximally contract more and more fibers. As athletes become stronger, they do not acquire new muscle fibers; instead, their nervous system learns to better use fibers and to employ previously unused fibers. The nervous system, however, only learns to do this by gradually overloading the muscles with more and more weight during each workout. This can be done with free-standing weights, expensive weight machines, or even bricks. Equipment is not the major determinant of strength development—effort is!

Emphasize the progressive aspects of the overload principle. Many coaches as well as some athletes become overzealous and overload too much, too quickly. It takes both time and nutrients for the body to recover from strength training sessions and to be able to recruit more and stronger muscle fibers. In fact, strength is actually gained between workouts, not during. If the body is not allowed 48 to 96 hours to recover between workouts as shown in Figure 9.1, muscular strength will actually decrease as illustrated in Figure 9.2. The remaining subprinciples should help you use the overload principle to design progressive strength training programs.

Use a long-term approach to strength development. Youngsters entering the sports world at the age of 8 or 9 can begin working on strength development, but with the idea of gaining only a little strength each year. Furthermore, the types of activities that will

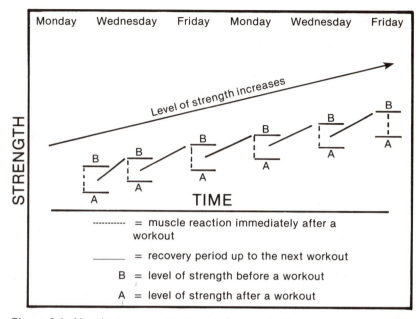

Figure 9.1. *Muscle recovery patterns before and after alternate day workouts. From D.P. Riley (Ed.),* Strength Training by the Experts. *West Point, NY: Leisure Press, 1977. Copyright 1977 by Leisure Press. Reprinted by permission.*

overload the muscles of an 8-year-old are considerably different than those for a high school athlete. Prepubescent athletes should use their body weight as the source of overload or resistance, but older athletes must provide greater resistance for the muscles by using any of many pieces of weight-training apparatus. For older athletes, simply moving the body during the execution of the sport or activity represents an "underload." Thus, as athletes become stronger, resistive devices such as weights and weight machines must be utilized to develop strength. (Some specific overload techniques for the various age groups will be given later in this chapter.)

Year-round programs are ideal for strength development. An intense, 3-week strength training program before the season begins only results in sore muscles and possible injuries. A less intense, long-term program will not only result in less muscle soreness but higher ultimate strength values, as shown in Figure 9.3. The long-term approach also helps athletes develop the exercise habit by having them involved on a regular basis. Successful long-term programs must vary the intensity of training and introduce "fun" activities into the strength training program.

Many athletes use strength training programs to increase muscle size

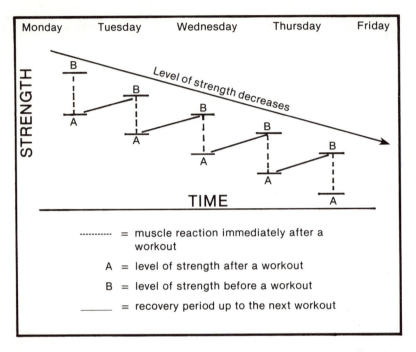

Figure 9.2. *Muscle recovery patterns before and after daily workouts. From D.P. Riley (Ed.),* Strength Training by the Experts. *West Point, NY: Leisure Press, 1977. Copyright 1977 by Leisure Press. Reprinted by permission.*

as well as strength. One caution, however: large gains in muscle size simply cannot be achieved by young boys before puberty or female athletes because neither of these groups have high enough levels of testosterone, the male hormone. Furthermore, many of the advanced lifting techniques and the tremendous loads used by professional football players and some field event performers to increase muscle size *cannot* and *should not* be attempted by younger athletes.

Vary the training frequency with the season. Frequency refers to the number of workouts per week. Leave 48-96 hours for muscles to recover in beginning and intermediate programs; that is, do training on 3 nonconsecutive days each week. If more than three quality workouts are squeezed into a week, the body simply will not be able to handle the stress; rather, athletes may lower their resistance, lose their appetite, lose weight, decrease their strength, and increase the possibility of stress fractures.

This training frequency should be used during the off-season and preseason periods; only 1-2 workouts should be used during the season. *Do not* stop the strength training during the season; doing so will result in the loss of the strength gains achieved during the preseason training. The 1 or 2 workouts will maintain athletes'

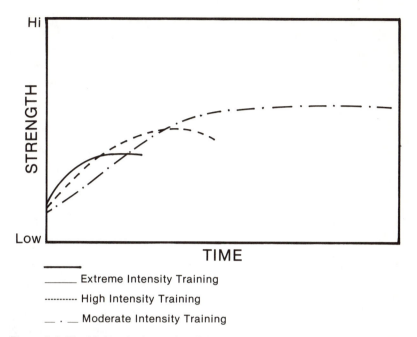

Figure 9.3. *The higher the intensity of the strength training, the faster improvement will be, but the peak strength values will not be as high as for those who take more time to develop strength.*

strength and still take up relatively little time from strategy and skill development.

The SAID Principle

The second major strength training principle is the SAID principle, or "Specific Adaptation to Imposed Demands." Translated, this means that if you want to improve the capacity of a particular muscle, that muscle must be identified and overloaded. If increased calf (gastrocnemius) and front thigh (quadriceps) strength is desired, then exercises which overload those muscles must be used. To apply this principle, you need to analyze the sport and the skills involved in your sport and decide which of the muscle groups are involved. Strength imbalances should also be analyzed for their potential contribution to injury. For instance, weak quadriceps and hamstrings, as well as quadriceps that are much stronger than the hamstrings, can cause knee injuries. Therefore, achieving a balance (about a 60:40 ratio) in quadricep and hamstring strength will help reduce the incidence of knee injuries as well as enhance performance.

Once the muscle groups and movements necessary for performing the sport's specific movements are identified, exercises can be selected to develop the muscles. This process can be somewhat simplified for coaches working with younger athletes, for at these younger ages (8-15), all athletes need to be developing the major muscle groups of the body. Consequently, a basic program should develop the following groups first before proceeding to more specialized exercises:

1. Quadriceps and gluteal muscles
2. Hamstrings
3. Gastrocnemius
4. Pectorals
5. Latissimus dorsi
6. Deltoids
7. Triceps
8. Biceps
9. Abdominal muscles
10. Muscles of spine area

Overload larger muscle groups before smaller ones. The larger muscle groups should be exercised before the smaller ones because smaller muscles tend to fatigue sooner and more easily than larger muscles. Thus, if the smaller muscles are fatigued, they may limit the intensity at which the athlete can work the larger muscles. Following this line of reasoning, a suggested exercise order would be:

1. Hips and lower back
2. Legs
   a. Quadriceps
   b. Hamstrings
   c. Calves
3. Trunk
   a. Upper back
   b. Shoulder
   c. Chest
4. Arms
   a. Triceps
   b. Biceps
   c. Forearms
5. Abdominals and spine
6. Neck

Although the abdominals and muscles of the spine are large muscle groups, they have been placed fifth because they function as stabilizers in most exercises. So, if high intensity work is performed early in the workout, with the abdominal and spine muscles, your athletes will find it difficult to exert maximal efforts during the other exercises.

Develop the muscles on both sides of a joint. All too frequently, strength training programs include quadricep work and no hamstring work or bicep exercises and no triceps exercises. For optimal flexibility and muscle balance for the prevention of injuries, exercise the muscles on one side of the joint and then on the other.

To follow this subprinciple, a basic strength training program should consist of the following core movements:

1. Hip and knee extension
2. Hip and knee flexion (especially leg curls)
3. Ankle flexion and extension
4. Shoulder and elbow extension
5. Shoulder and elbow flexion
6. Trunk flexion and extension and rotary movements (especially crunches, side bends, and bent trunk twists and trunk curls)

The specific exercises for these movements depend somewhat on the equipment available, but some examples using free weights and the Universal will be shown later.

Use the Repetition Maximum concept to establish the training intensity. The specificity principle not only has implications for which muscles should be exercised, but also for how hard they should be exercised, or in other words, how intense the training should be. Remember, although there must be an overload, athletes should not overwork their muscles. The Repetition Maximum or RM concept enables a training intensity to be prescribed so that the muscle is overloaded but not overworked by using the number of repetitions (the number of times an exercise is completed) as a way of specifying the resistance. Repetition Maximum is determined by the ability of the athlete to complete a prescribed number of exercises, meaning that optimal overload resistance is unique to each individual.

For example, a 6 RM is the amount of weight that an athlete can lift only six times. To allow for progress, usually an RM range is given. For instance, a 6-10 RM program means that the athlete finds the weight that can just barely be lifted six times with good form. Then he or she should continue to use that weight for that particular exercise until the muscles can lift the weight 10 times *with good form.* When this is possible, the athlete is ready to increase the overload. A good rule of thumb for increasing the overload is to use 1 additional pound for the upper body exercises for females, 2.5 lbs for upper body exercises for males, 5 lbs for lower body exercises for females, and 10 lbs for the lower body exercises for males.

Although a 6-10 RM range was used to illustrate the RM concept, research and practical experience have shown that by adjusting the exact RM numbers, the progressive adaptations of year-round programs for beginning and intermediate programs as well as the unique needs of certain types of athletes can be accommodated. For example, low repetition, high resistance work (6-10 RM) best develops muscle mass, whereas sets of more than 10 RMs tend to foster muscle endurance development. Increased muscle size and strength can be further enhanced by allowing for adequate recovery between sets (3-5 minutes). Conversely, muscle size gains can be *minimized* by supplementing low repetition, high resistance weight training with circuit training. Many successful training programs make such adjustments in RMs. The University of Nebraska, for instance, has two weight training programs. Those athletes (linemen, for example) who need to gain size and strength participate in high resistance work, whereas those players (backs and ends, for example) who need strength without large size gains combine circuit weight training with high resistance work. Because the idea of circuit training is to move quickly from station to station, the weight training time is greatly reduced.

Stop the exercise only when the muscle can no longer contract. When executing a set of 6-10 RMs, the set should not be ended just because the athlete completed 10 repetitions. The athlete should continue to try repetitions until the muscle groups can no longer contract. When the muscles can no longer contract, it is particularly effective to have a training partner who can not only urge the lifter on but also help the lifter get the weight up. Then the lifter can lower the weight. This is called "negative or eccentric work" and has been found to aid the overload process and facilitate strength gains.

Correct form should be maintained throughout the exercise. Once the specific exercises have been selected, you must teach athletes the correct form. Generally speaking, correct form means starting with as much stretch as possible on the muscle to be used and moving through the entire range of motion without fast, jerky movements to prevent the throwing of the weight. A good guide to follow is to lift the weight to a count of two and lower it to a count of four. The negative or lowering phase of the lift is important and should not be sacrificed by dropping the weight. Make sure your athletes control the lowering of the weight.

The exercise sequence should remain constant. If the exercises are completed in a different sequence each day, the muscles will be at different points of fatigue, causing the RM values to be wrong. By preparing a strength training record card similar to the one in Table 9.1, you can ensure that the exercise sequence is maintained and provide the athlete with an excellent source of feedback. Such feedback is important because strength training is the process of teaching the nervous system to recruit more muscle fibers and all learning occurs more rapidly with feedback. If improvements do not occur, the effort may have been insufficient or a change in routine may be indicated. Consequently, you may want to periodically change the exercises (not the muscle group) to relieve boredom and provide the spark for renewed gains.

Table 9.1

Strength Training Record

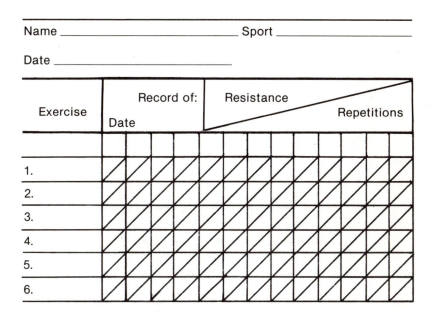

Name _____ Sport _____

Date _____

Exercise	Record of: Date	Resistance — Repetitions
1.		
2.		
3.		
4.		
5.		
6.		

The Principle of Reversibility

When athletes discontinue their strength training—i.e., when the overload is removed—the strength gains are gradually lost. The loss usually occurs more slowly than the gain, but nonetheless, strength will decrease if training is stopped during the season. If muscular strength is indeed important to performance and injury prevention, then strength training is just as important at the end of the season as at the beginning. Furthermore, because long-term strength development should be a goal, in-season strength maintenance programs will greatly enhance it, for as can be seen in Figure 9.4, in-season strength maintenance programs prevent strength losses and allow athletes to begin the off-season program at a higher level of strength development.

Designing the Strength Training Program

To develop a strength training program for your athletes, you need to integrate the principles just presented with some time and thought

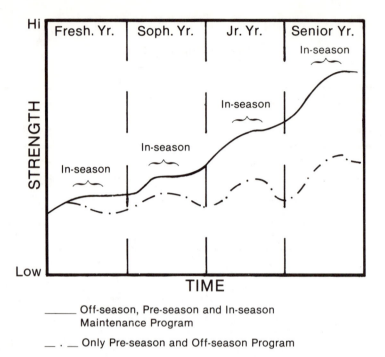

Figure 9.4. *In-season strength maintenance programs will greatly enhance the long-term strength development of athletes.*

to decide about the following:
1. Exercises to be performed;
2. Order of the exercises;
3. Number of repetitions to be performed (RM value);
4. Number of sets to be used;
5. Time interval between exercises; and
6. Number of workouts per week.

Many athletes know little about weight training principles or techniques. They think that as long as weight training causes them to sweat, they will improve. Therefore, take some time to explain the purposes of the program you have designed; it will be time well spent. Plan on taking several hours over 2 to 4 days to:

1. Explain the purposes of strength training in general;

2. Complete the necessary initial measurements. (Remember that in chapter 8, Table 8.2 presented some measurements to be used in evaluating weight gain. By taking these measurements before the strength training program is begun and periodically throughout the program you and the athlete will have some excellent feedback.)

3. Cover the safety rules to be used (see Table 9.2);

Table 9.2

Safety Rules for Training with Barbells

---

1. No horse play in the weight room.
2. Shoes, socks, and a shirt should be worn.
3. Make sure that the collars on each side of the barbell plates are tight and secure.
4. Use "spotters" to stand by and assist in positioning the weights and removing them. The spotters should also be motivators.
5. Do not hold your breath during the exercise. Exhale during the actual exertion.
6. Use a weightlifting belt when doing squats and dead lifts.

---

4. Discuss and demonstrate the individual exercises;

5. Point out why the individual exercises have been included, thus reinforcing why using the correct form is an absolute necessity;

6. Explain the use of the record card or sheet (see Table 9.1);

7. Allow the athletes to go through the program with the focus on learning techniques rather than seeing how much weight can be lifted (the younger the athlete, the longer this process).

Use these introductory sessions to assign training partners. Practical experience has shown that most people work hard and exert more effort when being urged on by a training partner. In addition, this individual or these individuals (if using free weights, two spotters are frequently needed) can help to complete the lifts during the final repetition(s), allowing the lifter to complete the negative work or eccentric phase of the lift.

Suggested Strength Training Activities for the Prepubertal Athlete

During the prepubertal years, the growth or epiphyseal plate of the long bones is still present; consequently, high intensity work against weights, weight machines, or isometric devices should be avoided because the extreme forces during this type of strength training may damage the growth plate. This does not mean that young athletes should forget strength training; it simply means that during these formative years, circuit training programs using timed calisthenics and light weights are more appropriate. Emphasize fun and fundamentals so youngsters enjoy participating. Strength training with weights or weight machines can be introduced as interest dictates, but the emphasis should be on learning safety procedures and correct techniques for the various exercises, *not* on how much weight can be lifted.

There are many possible circuit training combinations, so the following circuit should serve merely as an example. All circuits, however, should be organized to accommodate youngsters of varying abilities. Remember, to improve strength the muscles must be overloaded but not overworked, and because initial strength varies, you must individualize the training for each athlete.

Developing Calisthenic Circuit Training Programs

An exercise circuit is a series of 8 to 10 exercise stations which have been arranged so that the athlete can progress rapidly from one station to the next. You apply the SAID principle by selecting exercises which overload the major muscles used when performing. The overload is individualized by using exercise target numbers (the number of repetitions at a given station) and goal times (the amount of time in which an athlete will try to complete a trip through the circuit), and the number of trips through the circuit. The following sample directions should help you see how this information can be conveyed to your athletes.

Sample Directions

1. Explain all of the exercise stations (see Table 9.3) to the athletes. Point out that some stations have various "levels" of a given exercise, with Level I being the easiest.

2. Tell the youngsters that the first day's training will be to determine maximum capabilities. For instance, at Station 7 the youngster must determine which level sit-up he or she can do correctly. Then the youngster must try to see how many repetitions of sit-ups may be completed in a specified time (usually this is 1 minute). After recording this number have the athlete run to the next station and repeat the procedure with the new exercise.

3. To begin, have the athletes go to the stations. On the signal, have each youngster start, making sure he or she has the circuit training target-setting card (Table 9.4) to record in the "Max. # in 1 minute" column the maximums achieved at each station. You can use a stop watch to time the exercise period for each station. (Warning: If you do not have such a time limit, many of the exercises could be done at a slow pace for a very long time.)

4. After each youngster has completed all of the stations, the individual target exercise values are determined by halving the max-

Table 9.3

The Circuit Stations

Station 1: Squat Thrusts
— From a standing position, drop to a squat position. With the weight supported on the palms, thrust both legs out to extension and then draw them back in to the squat position. Stand up and repeat as many as possible in 1 minute.

Station 2: Springs
Level I - Obstacle 4 inches high
Level II - Obstacle 7 inches high
Level III - Obstacle 10 inches high
— While standing with the side to a rope (elastic ropes are nice because catching a foot does no damage) or other obstacle of the specified height, jump up and laterally over the obstacle. After a 2 foot landing, jump back across the obstacle. Try to complete as many as possible in 1 minute.

Station 3: Rope Climb
Level I - Climb with arms and legs
Level II - Arms only
Level III - Arms only with weight added
— Using a climbing rope that is 10-12 feet high, have the athletes climb up, climb down (controlled) and touch the floor with the right hand before starting the next ascent (do not touch floor with feet).

Station 4: Hop Kicks
— From a standing position jump up and kick heels together out to right side of body, land and repeat to left side. Continue to alternate sides.

Station 5: Side Lifts
— While lying on side with arms behind neck and legs extended, lift shoulders off the ground as high as possible, lower shoulders, roll to other side and repeat.

Table 9.3 (Cont.)

The Circuit Stations

Station 6: Push-ups

Level I - Modified (from knee)

Level II - Eccentric push-ups (start in regular push-up position and lower to a four-count cadence)

Level III - Regular push-ups

Level IV - Feet on a bench (the height of the bench may be varied for additional levels)

Level V - Handstand push-ups (use the wall to maintain balance

---

Station 7: Sit-ups (bent-knee)

Level I - Arms across chest

Level II - Hands clasped behind neck

Level III - Crunches (see Figure 9.18)

Station 8: Mountain Climbers or Treadmills

— Starting from the "up" position of regular push-ups, draw a knee up toward the chest simulating a running action (as if running up a very steep hill and the hands are being used to support body weight).

---

imum values. That is, if an athlete did 26 mountain climbers, his or her target number is 13. This number should be recorded on the circuit training target-setting card in the "Target #" column. The individual's starting station should also be marked (in the "Station #" column). This will establish the exercise sequence for that athlete. This arrangement will accommodate more youngsters because they will not all be starting at Station 1 simultaneously. You may elect to do the determining of the exercise target numbers for your younger athletes, but as the athletes get older they should share more and more of the responsibility for their training.

5. The goal time cannot be determined until the next time the group meets. At that time the athletes should go to their starting station. The purpose of this session is to determine how long it takes each youngster to complete two trips through the circuit, doing his or her target number of exercises for each station. By having a large clock or calling off the times, the completion time can be noted on the circuit training target-setting card.

Table 9.4

Circuit Training Target Setting Card

Name_____ Height_____ Weight_____

Age_____ Sport _____

Station #	Name of Exercise	Date_____ Max. # in 1 Minute	Exercise Target #	Date_____ Max. # in 1 Minute	Exercise Target #
	Squat thrusts				
	Log hops				
	Rope climb				
	Hop kicks				
	Side lifts				
	Push-ups				
	Sit-ups				
	Mountain climbers				

Goal time = _____ min.

6. The goal time is then found by taking ¾ of the actual time. Thus, if an athlete took 20 minutes to complete two circuit trips, the goal is to do the same amount of work in 15 minutes (20 × .75 = 15). When this goal is reached, the overload should be increased by lowering the time again (taking ½ of the original), adding a third trip through the circuit, redetermining the target number of exercises, or even changing the exercise stations.

7. You should keep the Target Setting Cards for your athletes and only use them in resetting the overload, but a daily record card such as the one in Table 9.5 should be used by the athletes. Because progress is

Table 9.5

Circuit Training Daily Record Card

Name _____ Goal Time _____

New Goal Time _____

New Goal Time _____

	Date	Time	Date	Time
1.				
2.				
3.				
4.				
5.				
6.				

measured by decreases in the amount of time taken for the circuit, you will need to emphasize correct form and technique.

Basic Strength Training Programs

As boys and girls continue their interest in a particular sport, the desire to improve will draw them to weight training. The benefits and satisfaction derived from early weight training experiences will have a big impact on their future training. Thus it is vital that you develop a good, basic strength training program that can serve the needs of all your athletes. To help you, we have presented two different basic programs in Table 9.6, one for use with free weights (barbells and dumbbells) and one for use with the Universal or similar weight machines. Each of these programs exercise the major muscle groups and involve the core exercises discussed in the SAID Principle.

During the off-season, as discussed in the Gradual Overload Principle, emphasis should be placed on the development of muscular

Table 9.6

**Core Exercises
with Different Resistive Exercise Equipment**

Muscles Used	Free Weights	Weight Machine
Gluteals/Lower back	Stiff-legged deadlift Fig. 9.5a	Hyperextension Fig. 9.5b
Quadriceps	Squat Fig. 9.6a	Knee extensions or leg press Fig. 9.6b
Hamstrings	Leg curls Fig. 9.7	Leg curls Fig. 9.7
Calves	Calf raise Fig. 9.8a	Toe presses Fig. 9.8b
Latissimus dorsi	Bent-over rowing or bent-arm pullover Fig. 9.9a & 9.9b	Chin-up or latissimus pulldowns Fig. 9.10
Trapezius	Shoulder shrug Fig. 9.11	Shoulder shrug Fig. 9.11
Deltoids	Upright rowing Fig. 9.12	Upright rowing Fig. 9.12
Pectoralis major	Bench press Fig. 9.13	Bench press or parallel dip Fig. 9.14
Biceps	Standing curls Fig. 9.15	Curls or chin-ups Fig. 9.15
Triceps	Triceps extensions with dumbbells Fig. 9.16a	Press down on 1st machine Fig. 9.16b
Forearms	Wrist curls Fig. 9.17	Wrist curls Fig. 9.17
Abdominals and spine area[a]	Sit-ups or crunches Fig. 9.18 Side bends with dumbbells Fig. 9.19 Trunk curls Fig. 9.21 Trunk twists Fig. 9.22	Sit-ups or crunches Fig. 9.18 Side bends Fig. 9.20 Trunk curls Fig. 9.21 Trunk twists (need a partner) Fig. 9.22
Neck[b]	Neck harness Fig. 9.23	Neck harness Fig. 9.23

[a]Essential for all young athletes
[b]For football and wrestling

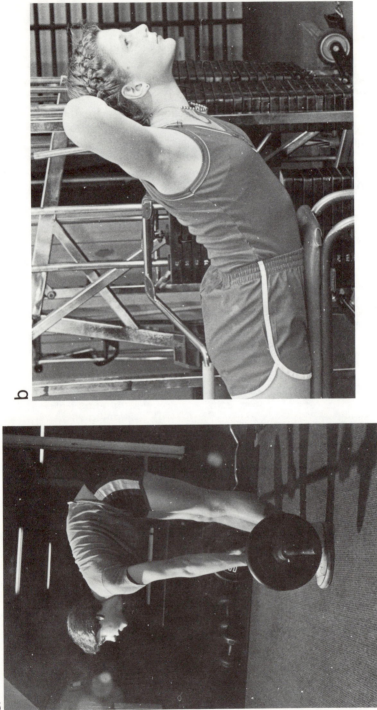

Figure 9.5. *Stiff-legged Dead Lift (a) and Hyperextensions (b)*

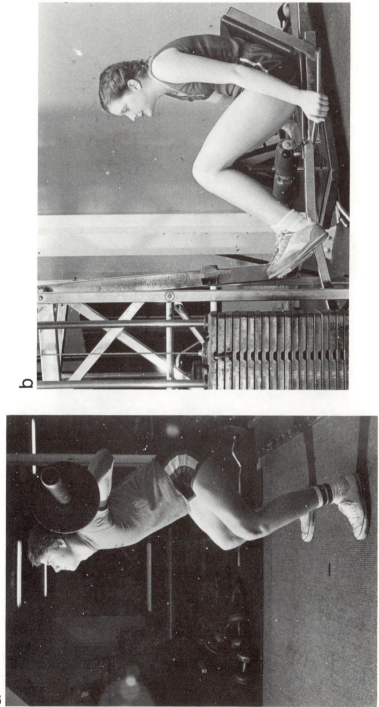

Figure 9.6. *Squat (a) and Leg Press (b)*

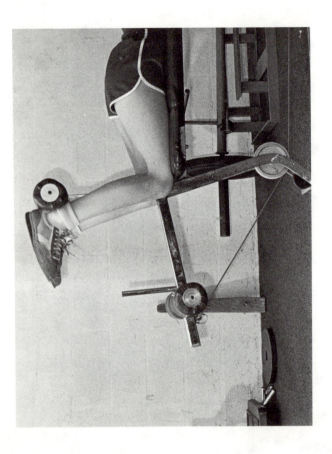

Figure 9.7. Leg Curls

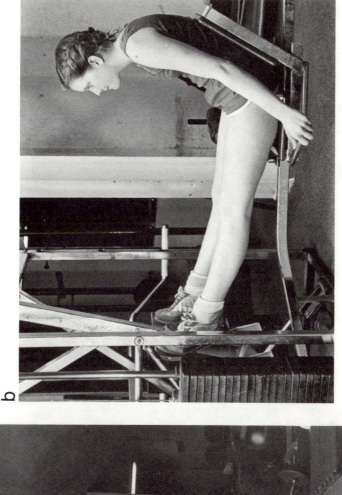

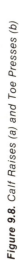

Figure 9.8. Calf Raises (a) and Toe Presses (b)

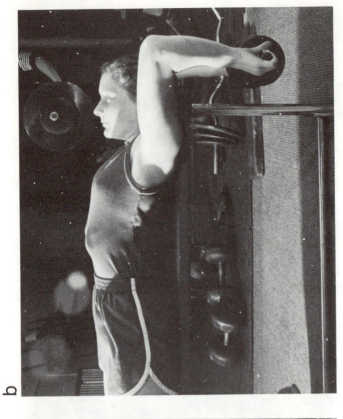

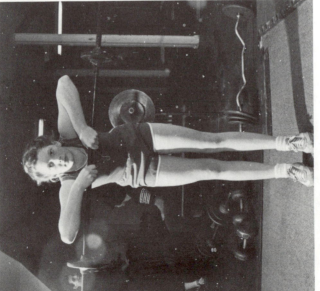

Figure 9.9. Bent-over Rowing (a) and Bent Arm Pullover (b)

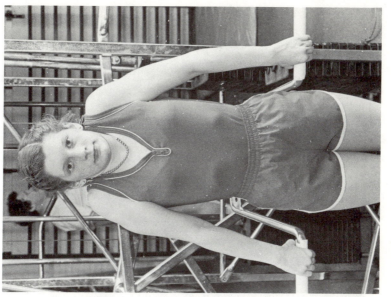

*Figure **9.11**. Shoulder Shrug*

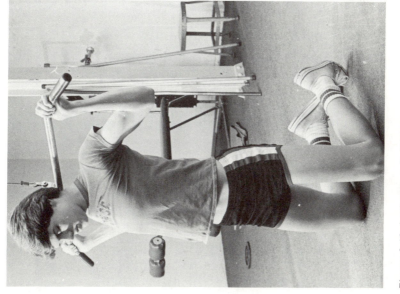

*Figure **9.10**. Latissimus Pulldown*

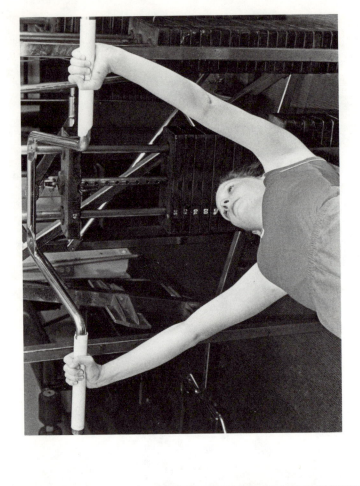

Figure 9.13. Bench Press

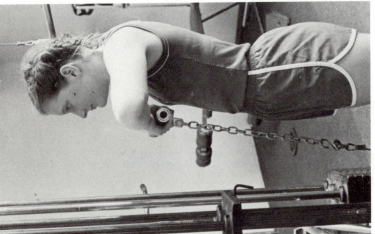

Figure 9.12. Upright Rowing

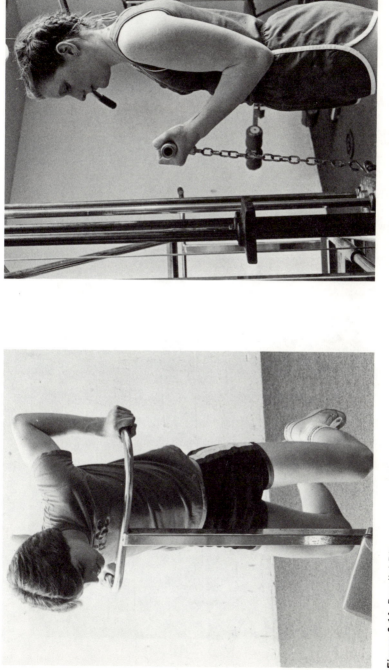

Figure 9.15. Standing Curls

Figure 9.14. Parallel Dip

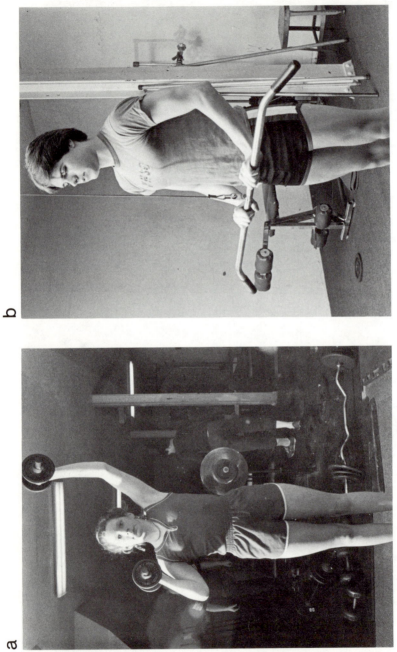

Figure 9.16. Triceps Extensions (a) and Press Downs (b)

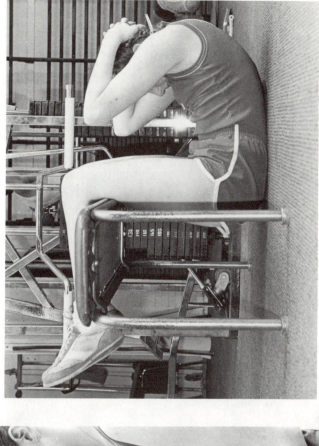

Figure 9.18. *Crunches*

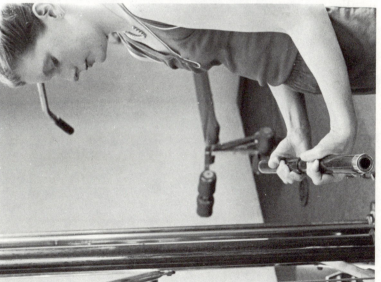

Figure 9.17. *Wrist Curls*

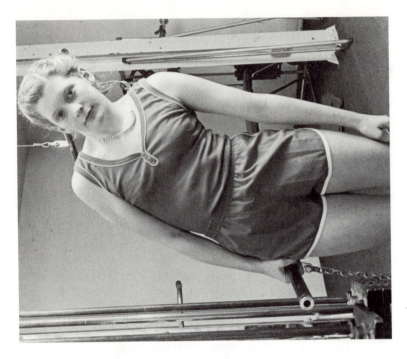

Figure 9.20. Side Bends

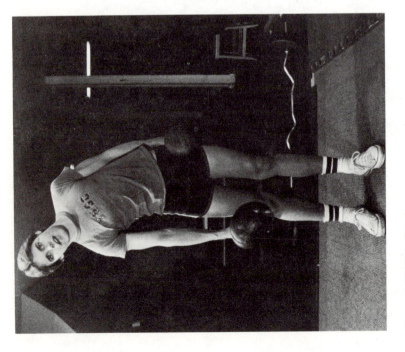

Figure 9.19. Side Bends

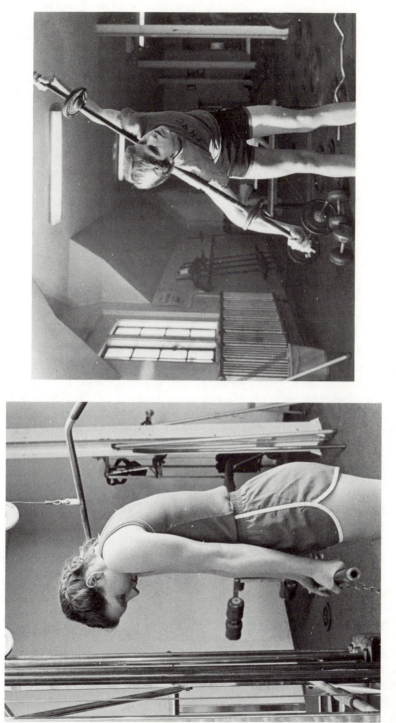

Figure 9.22. Trunk Twists

Figure 9.21. Trunk Curls

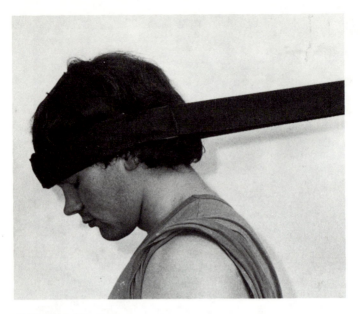

Figure 9.23. Neck Harness

strength by using one to three sets (one set for beginners and progressing to three) of 6-10 RMs. (For athletes younger than 13-14 years of age, 10-20 RMs with lighter weights is more appropriate.) Remember to allow ample recovery time—3 minutes between the various exercises and 5 minutes between sets. Then as the season approaches, the weight training can be completed using circuit training with 10-20 RMs and one to two trips through the circuit. Although the athlete is to move quickly through the circuit, this is accomplished by foregoing recovery time between lifts and sets and *not* by throwing the weights. The actual lifting style should not change.

Although your beginning and intermediate weight trainers may all be doing the same exercises, the maximum amount of weight that they can lift will vary from individual to individual. They should be aware of this and should not make comparisons between themselves. Comparisons with oneself are the only comparisons appropriate for weight training programs. The idea of strength training is to develop strength, not to see who can lift the most weight.

Not only should you tell your athletes that they all may be lifting different amounts of weight, but you should help them realize that not all people gain strength at the same rate or in the same manner. Some individuals have inherited muscles that are particularly well suited to developing strength and have very efficient lever systems due to the length of their bones and the muscle attachments to their bones. Similarly, the hormonal differences between males and females have considerable impact on the way muscle size develops in males and females. Several research studies have shown that through strength training, females can increase their relative strength values just as males do, but the females do not experience the same increase in muscle size (hypertrophy) as males.

Strength Training Programs for Girls and Women

The same major training principles that apply to males apply to females. We are not advocating that you design different programs for girls and women, but because society has treated females differently than males, special consideration needs to be given to certain aspects of program development.

Special time and consideration needs to be spent on developing a social and cultural environment conducive to girls becoming stronger. In other words, female athletes need to be exposed to an environment that allows both boys and girls to realize and accept that females are capable of doing long, hard work. For you this means:

1. Helping to inform hesitant parents about the myths surrounding females' participation in vigorous sports and the training that accompanies it. Either you can do this or you can arrange to have physicians, exercise physiologists, or other experts speak to the parents;

2. Debunking myths specifically about strength training being unfeminine and resulting in bulging muscles.

Advanced Weight Training for Weight Gain

During the later high school years, when the vulnerable bone growth plates have closed and athletes have had several years to become familiar with strength training techniques and procedures, an advanced program for the purpose of gaining size and *lean* weight as well as muscular strength can be implemented. In such a program, emphasis is placed on heavy resistive loads. Particular attention should be given to maximizing the effort exerted in the exercises which use the largest muscles of the body because they have the greatest potential for increase in size. Because maximizing the effort means working against heavy resistance, the number of repetitions must be relatively small. The following sample routine illustrates these points and therefore constitutes a good (training) program for gaining both strength and lean weight:

1. Squat: 1 set, 15 repetitions (warm-up); 5 sets, 6-8 repetitions
2. Bench press: 1 set, 15 repetitions; 5 sets, 4-6 repetitions
3. Bent rowing: 1 set, 15 repetitions; 5 sets, 6-8 repetitions
4. Bent-arm pullover: 3 sets, 12-15 repetitions

5. Two hand curls: 3 sets, 6-8 repetitions
6. Dead lift: 1 set, 15 repetitions; 3 sets, 8-10 repetitions
7. Leg curls: 3 sets, 6-10 repetitions
8. Side bends: 3 sets, 6-10 repetitions
9. Bent trunk twists: 3 sets, 6-10 repetitions
10. Sit-ups: 1 set, 15-20 repetitions (with extra resistance)

Only one set of sit-ups is included because excessive abdominal work seems to thwart weight gain. Only the resistance used should be increased gradually, not the number of sets or repetitions. At the conclusion of this program, the athlete should be unable to do any more work. If the athlete feels capable of continuing, heavier resistance should be used next time. Heavy resistive exercise programs, such as the one just described, will result in substantial strength gains for all athletes, but the gains in lean weight will be much more variable. Remember, gaining lean weight is contingent on not only working against heavy resistance but also on eating properly, getting enough sleep, and having the right body type and androgen levels.

You can use the training principles presented in this chapter to design the heavy resistive work, and the information on gaining lean weight from chapter 8 to help athletes adjust their caloric intake and ensure adequate protein consumption, but you can't do anything about the athlete's genetic endowment. Many athletes, including most women, simply do not have the potential to develop massive musculature. It is very important that your athletes realize this so they do not become discouraged if they are not gaining weight and increasing their muscle girths. It is far more important that the athletes increase their muscular strength than muscle bulk, so use the feedback from the daily strength training records and periodic strength tests to reinforce this. And perhaps most importantly, use the skinfold caliper and the waist and girth measurement every 2-3 weeks to evaluate body fat. The triceps and subscapular skinfold thicknesses, as well as the waist girth, should not increase. This is an especially critical concept to convey to athletes gaining weight. They must realize that "bigger is not necessarily better" if the weight gain is due to an increased amount of body fat.

Summary

Helping your athletes to adopt nutritionally sound eating habits and calorie-burning exercise habits will certainly help them reduce body fat, but in order to develop lean tissue, athletes need to engage in strength training. Therefore, we encourage you to promote strength training as an integral part of your physical and nutritional conditioning programs.

Chapter 10
The High-Octane Diet

The High-octane Diet, sometimes called carbohydrate loading or glycogen packing, is designed to provide optimal quantities of high-energy fuel foods. This is not a weight loss diet. It is an eating plan designed to optimize performance by making adequate energy fuels available to the muscles and nerves. It is not a substitute for training, practice, and weight control. Thus, we are not including this chapter to indicate that food is a substitute for lean, fit, and skilled performers, but that the content of the meals in the days prior to competition can influence athletic performance. The High-octane Diet should only be used after you and perhaps the team physician have agreed upon an ideal weight according to the guidelines presented in chapter 2 and after this ideal weight has been properly obtained.

The High-octane Diet is the culmination of much research. This research taught us that dietary carbohydrates are broken down into simple sugars (glucose) which are taken into the muscle and liver cells and stored as glycogen. When involved in high intensity, strenuous physical activities such as in wrestling or gymnastics, the

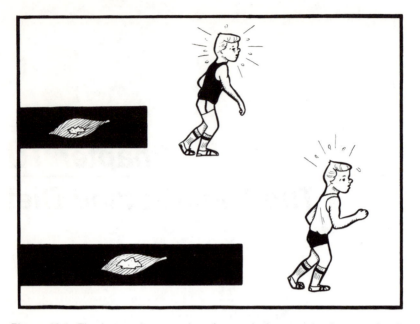

Figure 10.1. *The larger the quantity of stored glycogen in the muscle, the longer physical activity can be sustained.*

muscle cells can then burn the stored glucose molecules and release the necessary energy. In addition, the liver cells can release their stored glucose into the blood, thus ensuring the nerve tissues a continuous supply of glucose for fuel. Because glucose is the preferred fuel for muscles during strenuous activities, researchers have theorized that the supply of glucose that can be stored in the muscles sets the limits for physical activity. In other words, if only a small supply of glucose is stored in the muscle, that muscle will not be able to contract vigorously for as long as would be possible if a larger supply had been stored.

A series of studies by a team of Swedish physiologists verified this theory. In these studies, a muscle biopsy procedure was used to sample muscle tissue prior to and after exercise. In this manner, they were able to observe that there was indeed a relationship between the amount of glycogen stored in a muscle and that muscle's capacity for vigorous physical activity. The greater the concentration of glycogen in the muscle before exercise, the longer the activity could be sustained until exhaustion.

"Can the amount of glycogen stored in the muscle be regulated by manipulating the diet?" was the obvious next question. It was found that while on a normal diet the average concentration of glycogen in the muscle tissues was approximately 1.75 grams per 100 grams of

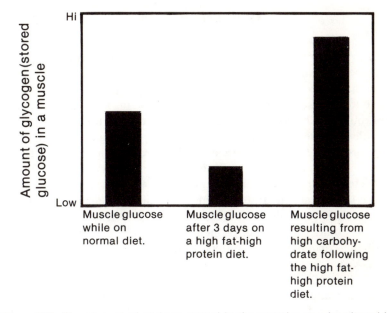

Figure 10.2. *The amount of glucose stored in the muscles can be altered by diet.*

muscle. After 3 days of a diet limited to fat and protein (with carbohydrates entirely eliminated), the glycogen level fell to 0.6 grams per 100 grams of muscle. This dietary protocol was then reversed and large amounts of carbohydrates were added to the menu. Now when muscle biopsies were taken, the glycogen stored in the muscle increased substantially (3.5 grams/100 grams of muscle). These changes in the glycogen stored in the muscles are shown in Figure 10.2. The foundation for the High-octane Diet is based on this finding.

Because sports differ in the rate and the length of time in which energy is being used, the amount of fuel necessary for optimal energy varies for different sports. Thus slightly different high-octane eating plans have been developed to meet the specific needs of sports with different energy demands. Three versions or modifications of the High-octane Diet are presented to meet the needs of these different sports. High-octane Plan 1 is for athletes involved in endurance events lasting longer than 1 hour (distance running, swimming, and cross country skiing). High-octane Plan 2 is most appropriate for sports intense in nature, particularly if the activity is repeated several times such as in a tournament. High-octane Plan 3 is also intended for activities that are intense in nature, the only differences in Plan 2 and Plan 3 being that the first phase of Plan 2 is dropped.

High-octane Plan 1

Each of the three high-octane eating plans covers a 6-day period. Let's begin Plan 1 on the Sunday before a Friday evening event. Phase 1 of the plan, which lasts for 2½ to 3 days, begins with an initial depletion workout followed by a diet of proteins and fats. This initial workout must be 90 minutes in duration and very intense. Its purpose is to deplete the body's quick energy stores, leaving the athlete feeling very tired. The athlete then eats a high protein-high fat diet for the next 2½ to 3 days. The daily carbohydrate consumption must be restricted to approximately 100 grams or 400 Calories a day during Phase 1. The carbohydrate content of the diet can be monitored fairly accurately by consulting the information in Appendix D. This information could then be supplemented with one of the commercially available carbohydrate counters which you can find at your local bookstore.

In Tables 10.1, 10.2, and 10.3, we present information for planning meals that might be consumed during Phase 1. The exact caloric consumption per day depends on the size of the athlete and his or her daily physical activities (see chapters 7 and 8). For example, if the athlete expends 3,000 Calories a day, including training and practice, then Phase 1 of the High-octane Plan 1 should consist of 2,700 to 3,000 Calories. The majority of the 2,700 to 3,000 Calories consumed daily should come from those foods high in fat and protein (see Table 10.2). The carbohydrate content of the diet during Phase 1 should be limited to 100-110 grams (400-440 kcal) per day and should be selected from the cereal and fruit groups, not junk foods.

During Phase 1, the athlete should be continuing to work out or train vigorously. This combination of hard work and low carbohydrate intake will deplete the glycogen stores in the liver and muscles. Consequently, the athlete will feel a little tired and will have to push to train. This sense of fatigue is not unusual, for the body is having to use fat rather than sugar as an energy source. You should prepare your athletes for the fatigue by explaining why they will feel tired and cautioning them not to defeat the purpose of Phase 1 by stuffing themselves with junk foods.

By Wednesday or after 2½-3 days, the athlete should begin Phase 2. During Phase 2, the diet should still contain adequate protein and fat, but the carbohydrate content can be increased. The total caloric consumption, however, should not exceed the maintenance level of calories. The idea is to maximally over "fill" the sugar or glycogen reserves of the muscles, not to gorge the athlete. Thus, low residue (low bulk) carbohydrate sources, such as those listed in Table 4.2, are recommended. This procedure results in a greater than normal storage

Table 10.1

**The High-octane Diet
for Maximizing Muscle Glycogen Stores**

	PHASE 1	PHASE 2
Protein and fat sources (like meat, eggs, milk, butter, sour cream)	55-65% of the kcal (4-5 servings)	10% of the kcal (1-2 servings)
Low calorie, high bulk vegetables and fruits (cucumbers, tomatoes, celery, carrots, etc.)	10-20% of the kcal	Minimize because of the bulk
Bread, cereals, vegetables, and fruits	20% of the kcal or at least 400 kcal per day	70-80% of the kcal
Desserts	Nonsweetened gelatin	10-15% of the kcal (but avoid junk foods)
Beverages	As much nonsugared fluid as desired (At least 1 liter of water for every 1,000 kcal)	As much as desired as long as caloric balance is maintained

of glycogen, allowing distance runners or swimmers to work hard for a longer period of time. It does *NOT* allow them to run or swim faster, only maintain their speed longer.

Phase 3 of the High-octane Diet is the same for all three plans and centers on the consumption of an appropriate pre-event meal. Sports in general are frequently steeped in mythology and superstitions. Socks are not washed once a winning streak begins, certain shirts are lucky, and many pregame or pre-event procedures have become rituals. This is particularly true of the pre-event meal. For example, the proverbial steak has almost become as much a part of American football lore as the roll of the drums for the kick-off. Nevertheless, let's leave mythology and look a bit more scientifically at the pre-event meal.

Energy consumption should be sufficient to prevent feelings of

Table 10.2

The High Fat-High Protein Diet

What you CAN eat during Phase 1

MEAT
Almost any kind of beef, pork, or lamb, including spareribs, corned beef, lamb chops, tongue, hamburgers, roast veal. (Sausage, hot dogs, and packaged cold cuts with filler must be avoided, however.)

FOWL
All forms of chicken, turkey, duckling, and other fowl.

SEAFOOD
Any kind of fish or seafood—including shrimp, lobster, oil-packed tuna and smoked salmon—except oysters, clams, mussels, scallops, and pickled fish.

DAIRY PRODUCTS
Eggs in any style, 4 ounces a day of any hard cheese (no cream cheese or spreads), 4 teaspoons a day of heavy cream (no milk—it has more carbohydrates), and unlimited quantities of butter and other fats.

BEVERAGES
Unlimited amounts of water, mineral water, club soda, beef or chicken broth, bouillon, sugar-free diet soda, and tea. Coffee should be limited to six cups a day. You can also have the juice of one lemon or lime, but not orange juice.

GREEN SALADS
Two small (less than 1 cup) salads a day, made of the following ingredients: cabbage (regular or Chinese), celery, chicory, chives, cucumber, endives, escarole, fennel, lettuce, olives (green or black), onions, pickles (sour or dill), parsley, peppers, radishes, scallions, watercress.

DRESSINGS AND GARNISHES
Oil and vinegar, Roquefort, and Caesar dressings. You can also add crumbled bacon, anchovies, fried pork rinds, grated cheese, minced hard-cooked egg, mushrooms, and even sour cream.

VEGETABLES
Asparagus, avocado, bamboo shoots, bean sprouts, beet greens, broccoli, brussels sprouts, cabbage, cauliflower, chard, Chinese cabbage, eggplant, kale, kohlrabi, mushrooms, okra, onions, peppers, pumpkin, rhubarb, sauerkraut, snow pea pods, spinach, string beans, summer squash, tomatoes, turnips, water chestnuts, wax beans, zucchini squash.

continued

CONDIMENTS
Salt, pepper, prepared or dry mustard, horseradish, vinegar, vanilla and other extracts, artificial sweeteners, any dry herb or spice containing no sugar.

DESSERTS
Limit desserts to fruits and unsweetened gelatins, but no more than 4 servings per day (total of 400 calories per day).

What you should not eat during Phase 1

FRUITS
Apples, bananas, dates, figs, dried fruits, grapes, oranges, raisins, yogurt with fruit (except as stated under desserts).

VEGETABLES
Beans (except wax and green), carrots, corn, peas, potatoes, sweet pickles, yams, rice.

BEVERAGES
Milk, soft drinks containing sugar, fruit juices (except unsweetened juice of one lemon or lime), milkshakes, tomato juice, V-8 juice.

BREADS AND CEREALS
Bread, cereals, spaghetti, macaroni, crackers.

OTHERS
Cashews, catsup, chewing gum, cookies, cornstarch, flour, honey, ice cream, jam, pancakes, pies, relish, sugar, syrup.

For the High-carbohydrate Diet, the foods on this "cannot" list are excellent. In addition, the High-Carbohydrate Diet can include:

MEAT
Sausage, hot dogs, and packaged cold cuts with filler are all high in carbohydrates.

SEAFOOD
Oysters, clams, mussels, scallops, and pickled fish.

DAIRY PRODUCTS
Cream cheese and spreads, milk (homogenized).

---

hunger or weakness prior to and during the competitive event. Although it is true that it takes several days to adequately fill muscle energy stores, the pre-event meal does play a significant role in altering the liver's sugar stores. These stores are in turn a very important fuel source for the athlete's nerves, but large meals are not necessary to ensure adequate energy. Rather, the pre-event meal should be low in residue, contain familiar foods, avoid gas-producing foods, and be eaten 3-4 hours before competition.

Table 10.3

Sample Meal Plans

PHASE 1	PHASE 2
Breakfast	**Breakfast**
8 oz tomato juice 4 eggs 1 slice toast 4 tsp butter or margarine 4 strips bacon	8 oz orange juice (sweetened or unsweetened) 1 egg 2 slices toast 2 tsp butter or margarine 1 cup cereal
Lunch	**Lunch**

1 serving meat
2-3 cheese sticks
1 tossed salad with oil dressing
1 medium apple or orange
	2 sandwiches—each with 1 oz
	  meat or cheese, ½ tsp butter
	  or margarine
	8 oz lowfat milk
	2 large bananas

Snack(s)	**Snack(s)**
Meat 1 cheese stick 1 medium apple or banana	2 sandwiches—meat or nonmeat 1 serving fruit 8 oz lowfat milk
Dinner	**Dinner**

10 oz meat (not ham)
1 serving vegetable (no corn,
etc.) with 1-2 tsp butter or
margarine and sour cream
1 tossed salad
1 small apple
D-Zerta
	4 oz meat (not ham)
	1 medium baked potato, with 1
	tsp butter, etc.
	1 serving vegetable
	2 rolls, with 1 tsp butter or
	  margarine
	2 servings fruit
	2 servings beverage, such as
	  Hy-Cal or Cal-power

Some athletes have particularly nervous stomachs and gastrointestinal tracts; consequently a liquid prematch meal might be appropriate for them. Several of these commercial liquid meals are available, each of which is high in carbohydrate content and contains sufficient fat and protein to give a satisfied feeling and relieve hunger. Athletes who are not familiar with liquid meals should experiment with them prior to actually using them before competition. *The prematch meal is no time to be trying new fads.*

Although the concept of using liquids to optimize the body's prematch energy stores is important, the role of "liquid energy meals" is probably even more important to athletes involved in a tournament. Under such circumstances, athletes frequently perform several times in 1 day. Thus, the liquid meal provides a quick way of replenishing the body's energy stores. The low residue foods listed in Table 4.2 do so as well.

Remember, however, that although liquid formulas may have a place in the prematch preparations, their use should not be extended to daily consumption. First of all, they are expensive. In addition, using them daily does not allow athletes to practice planning a nutritionally sound diet. Last, the gastrointestinal tract needs to handle a certain amount of bulk or fiber—which liquid meals lack—or it becomes very sluggish.

Another precaution is to refrain from adding extra protein or carbohydrate to the liquid meals. Doing so can produce severe cramping and diarrhea because of the unusually high concentrations of protein or carbohydrate in "doctored" liquid meal preparations. Once again, "if a little is good, a lot is not necessarily better." The stomach simply cannot handle extremely concentrated drinks. Similar complications have arisen from "doctored" commercially available breakfast substitutes or reducing formulas.

High-octane Plan 2

Many sports and activities do not require athletes to run, swim, or cycle for 2-3 continuous hours. Therefore, the need to overfill the muscle glycogen "storage tanks" is not so great. Also, some athletes are unable to train following the 90-minute depletion period discussed in Plan 1. But sports such as basketball, volleyball, soccer, gymnastics, and football do require numerous bouts of intense activity, so having the liver and muscle glycogen storage tanks filled is desirable, even if they are not overfilled.

To accomplish this, Plan 2 leaves out the preceding plan's 90-minute period of intense exercise for depleting glycogen stores. Instead the training and practice takes place as usual, and the high fat-high protein diet described in Tables 10.1 and 10.2 is followed.

After 2½-3 days of Phase 1, athletes should change to Phase 2, which is a high carbohydrate diet. Remember to warn your athletes that just because they are increasing the percentage of their total calories eaten as carbohydrates does not mean that they should gorge

Table 10.4

Foods High in Salt

Anchovies	Kale
Bacon	Kosher meat
Barbecue sauce	Meat tenderizer
Beans, butter	Mustard
Beans, dried lima	Olives
Bologna and other	Peanut butter
luncheon meats	Pickles
Bouillon	Potato chips and corn chips
Bread and rolls	Pretzels
(especially those	Relishes
with salt topping)	Salt pork
Catsup	Salted nuts
Cheese, American	Salted popcorn
Cheese, Swiss	Salty and smoked fish
Cheese, cheddar	Salty and smoked meat
Chili sauce	Sardines
Chipped and corned beef	Sauerkraut
Cottage cheese	Sausage
Crackers	Seasonings (salt,
Diet pop	monosodium glutamate,
Dry cereals	poultry seasoning, etc.
French fries	Soups (canned)
Ham	Soy sauce
Herring	Tuna and other canned fish
Horseradish	Vegetables (canned)
Hot dogs	Worcestershire sauce

themselves. Caloric balance for weight control is still necessary, so again low residue, high carbohydrate foods are appropriate.

Plan 2 of the High-octane Diet also is particularly well suited for sports which have weight classes, such as wrestling and crew, because Phase 2 of this plan calls for a restriction on high bulk and salty foods. To help you implement these restrictions, we have listed some foods in Table 10.4 which should be removed from the athletes' diet in the 72 hours prior to the contest. (See Table 4.2 for some suggested high energy, low residue foods.) By removing bulky or high residue foods from the Phase 2 diet, athletes minimize the food residue present in the bowel. This is helpful for the "weigh-in" for wrestlers and enhances the performance of all athletes.

Note, however, that the bowel should not be emptied at the expense

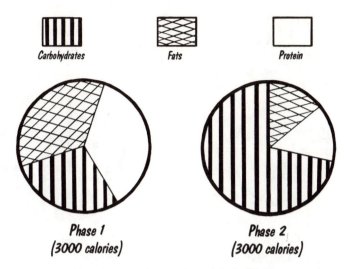

Figure 10.3. *For most athletes, the number of Calories consumed on a daily basis may be quite constant, but the proportion of fats, proteins, and carbohydrates consumed should vary as the week progresses.*

of precious body water as with laxatives. In fact, to ensure adequate hydration, have your athletes consume at least eight full glasses of water every day during the 72 hours prior to the competition. Because the salt intake is being curtailed, little of this water will be retained. Thus, drinking water will not increase body weight.

By now it should be evident that the concept of the High-octane Diet is not based on the magical properties of some special wonder foods; rather it is just the application of sound nutritional and physiological factors. Consequently, these high octane dietary suggestions may have to be modified to meet the individual needs of athletes. For example, some individuals have a very difficult time tolerating the low carbohydrate consumption of Phase 1, so for these individuals, Plan 3 may be used.

High-octane Plan 3

This modification of the High-octane Diet merely consists of increasing the number of carbohydrate Calories in Phase 1 to a more tolerable level. If the athlete is too tired and out of sorts to practice, attend classes, or get along with family and peers, the restriction on carbohydrate consumption should be removed or reestablished at a higher level (400 to 600 grams or 1,600 to 2,400 kcal). Furthermore, recent research seems to indicate that the "super-loading" effects of

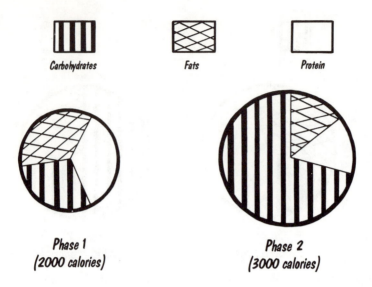

Figure 10.4. *During the High-octane Diet, the total number of Calories consumed on a daily basis may be somewhat lower at the beginning of the week
than later in the week. Even more importantly, the percentage of carbohydrates consumed changes as the week progresses.*

carbohydrate restriction loses its impact if done every week. Consequently, Plans 1 and 2 of the High-octane Diet should be restricted to
just once or twice a year or for special competitive events. Also, the
psychological impact of the High-octane Diet may be enhanced if the
high protein-high fat part of the diet is used only on a limited basis.

In addition, some individual variability may have to be employed in
terms of establishing the daily caloric consumption schedule. For
some, it may be best to keep the daily caloric consumption value about
equal and merely alter the composition of the Calories during Phase 1
and Phase 2 as illustrated in Figure 10.3. For others, it may be more
desirable to restrict the number of Calories consumed early in the
week and increase the number of Calories consumed as the day of
competition arrives. Such a procedure is illustrated in Figure 10.4.
Either of these procedures is appropriate and should be accomplished
without allowing more than a 3-pound weekly fluctuation in the
athlete's weight. For if athletes' weight is allowed to ''bounce'' up and
down by more than 3 pounds from week to week, they are using shifts
in body water to control weight. Consequently, they are running the
risk of impairing performance potentials by depriving muscles of
necessary water. Knowing this, you will be in a better position to prevent your athletes from using the ''roller coaster'' approach to weight
control.

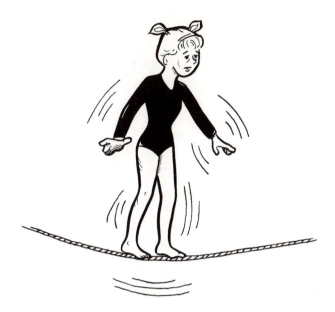

Figure 10.5. *Don't let your athletes walk a weight control tightrope. Help them with a sound nutritional conditioning program.*

Summary

The meals and snacks that athletes eat in the days immediately prior to competition can influence their performance. Athletes who have optimal levels of muscle and liver glycogen and water will have the energy necessary to work vigorously throughout the competitive event. Consequently, your athletes' nutritional conditioning can be completed with the three high-octane dietary plans. Knowing this, you can help athletes and their parents plan meals and snacks to maximize competition energy levels without jeopardizing weight control.

Chapter 11
As the Caliper Turns

Athletes need not starve themselves and form poor nutritional habits. Rather, you can readily help your athletes avoid these pitfalls by:

1. Determining their ideal weight based on individual body composition;

2. Applying the weight loss or gain guidelines prior to the beginning of the competitive season to enable them to obtain their ideal weight;

3. Encouraging them to maintain their ideal weight throughout the season by planning a nutritional diet and balancing their caloric consumption and expenditure;

4. Incorporating strength training with your program;

5. Optimizing performance potentials by encouraging them to use the High-octane Diet and pre-event meal suggestions.

If you do each of these, your athletes should be able to have safe, successful, and enjoyable seasons. Furthermore, if you are able to convey to your athletes the weight control practices and dietary knowledge presented in this book, they will be forming valuable lifetime nutritional habits. They will learn that caloric consumption must not exceed caloric expenditure. They will learn to minimize salt intake. And finally, they will learn to eat balanced nutritional meals.

But these outcomes will only occur if you are able to get your athletes to adopt sound nutritional and weight control practices. The use of the behavior modification strategies mentioned in chapter 7 and various motivational and reward systems may help in this regard, but perhaps the most important tool can be found in the words of Edgar A. Guest.

I'd rather see a sermon than hear one any day;
I'd rather one should walk with me than merely tell the way.
The eye's a better pupil and more willing than the ear,
Fine counsel is confusing, but example's always clear;
And the best of all the preachers are the men who live their creeds,
For to see good put in action is what everybody needs.
I soon can learn to do it if you'll let me see it done;
I can watch your hands in action, but your tongue too fast may run.
And the lecture you deliver may be very wise and true,
But I'd rather get my lessons by observing what you do;
For I might misunderstand you and the high advice you give,
But there's no misunderstanding how you act and how you live.

From *Collected Verse of Edgar A. Guest*, p. 509. Copyright 1934 by Reilly & Lee Co. (now Contemporary Books). Reprinted with permission.

If you believe that optimal body composition fosters optimal performance, then turn the caliper on yourself to see if extra fat pounds are detracting from your health and efficiency. Have a fellow coach take your triceps skinfold, biceps skinfold, subscapular skinfold, and suprailiac skinfold. Remember, the accuracy of these tests depends upon locating the precise site for the skinfold and using the caliper correctly. Review chapter 2 for the instructions on using the caliper before you begin.

All of these measurements are to be taken on the right side. The triceps skinfold is taken over the triceps muscle at the point exactly halfway between the elbow (olecranon process) and the shoulder (acromion process) (see Figure 2.4 and Figure 2.6). Next, Figures 2.8 and 2.9 will help you locate the subscapular skinfold. Then take the biceps skinfold over the midpoint of the biceps muscle halfway between the shoulder and the elbow, as shown in Figures 11.1 and 11.2. Finally, take the suprailiac skinfold at the oblique fold of skin just above the hip bone (iliac crest). Use Figures 11.3 and 11.4 to locate the correct site.

After recording three measurements for each of the four locations on a recording form like that shown in Table 11.1, find the average for each location and then add these averages to determine the total skinfold value. Find the number in the "skinfold" column of Table 11.2

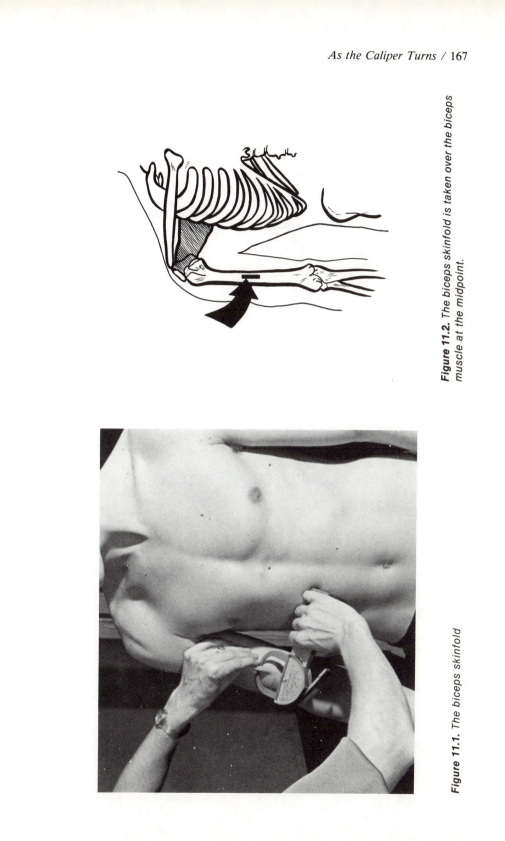

Figure 11.2. *The biceps skinfold is taken over the biceps muscle at the midpoint.*

Figure 11.1. *The biceps skinfold*

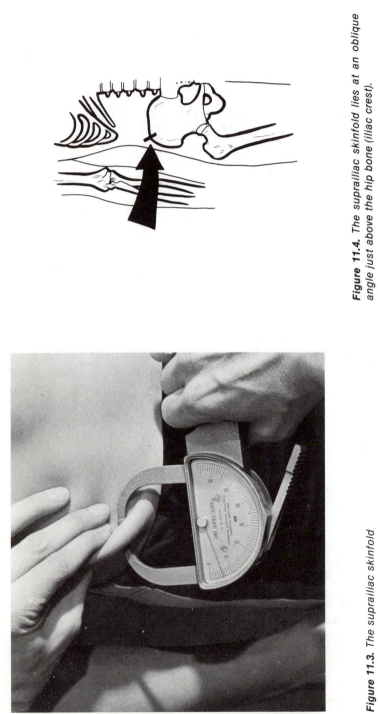

Figure 11.4. *The suprailiac skinfold lies at an oblique angle just above the hip bone (iliac crest).*

Figure 11.3. *The suprailiac skinfold*

Table 11.1

Body Composition Prediction for Males and Females
Seventeen Years and Above

Name _____ Date _____

Body Weight _____lbs   Sex _____

Ideal Percent Fat _____   Predicted Percent Fat _____

Lean Body Weight _____ lbs   Ideal Body Weight _____lbs

Skinfolds

	#1	#2	#3	Average
Triceps	_____ mm	_____ mm	_____ mm	_____ mm
Subscapular	_____ mm	_____ mm	_____ mm	_____ mm
Biceps	_____ mm	_____ mm	_____ mm	_____ mm
Suprailiac	_____ mm	_____ mm	_____ mm	_____ mm
			Total	_____ mm

Males

1. LBW = Body Weight − (% Fat × Body Weight)

    LBW = _____ lbs − (_____ × _____ lbs)

    _____ lbs = _____ lbs − (_____ lbs)

2. Ideal Weight = $\dfrac{\text{LBW}}{(100\% - \text{Ideal \% Fat})}$

    Ideal Weight = $\dfrac{\rule{3cm}{0.4pt}}{(1.00 - .16)}$

    _____ lbs = $\dfrac{\text{lbs}}{.84}$

    _____ lbs = _____

_____ continued _____

Table 11.1 (Cont.)

**Body Composition Prediction for Males and Females
Seventeen Years and Above**

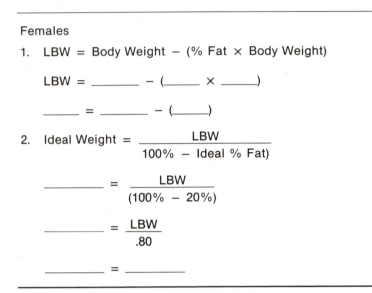

Females

1. LBW = Body Weight − (% Fat × Body Weight)

   LBW = _____ − (_____ × _____)

   _____ = _____ − (_____)

2. Ideal Weight = $\dfrac{\text{LBW}}{100\% - \text{Ideal \% Fat)}}$

   _____ = $\dfrac{\text{LBW}}{(100\% - 20\%)}$

   _____ = $\dfrac{\text{LBW}}{.80}$

   _____ = _____

that is closest to the skinfold total you just calculated. From this point in the skinfold column draw an imaginary straight line out to the right until you intersect the column which is appropriate for your sex and age. The value in this column will be your predicted percent fat. To find your ideal body weight, use the general formula

$$\text{Ideal Weight} = \frac{\text{Lean Body Weight}}{100\% - \text{Ideal \% Fat}}$$

and 16% fat as the ideal for adult males and 20% as the ideal value for adult females. (These ideal percent fat values are higher than those given for athletes because the average person is not trying to achieve maximal efficiency as is an athlete.) For example, if a 30-year-old male coach who weighs 200 lbs has a skinfold total of 100mm, his percent fat will be 29 and he will be about 32 lbs over his "ideal weight" of 168. (The sample calculations in Table 11.3 illustrate how the general formula is used to determine this ideal weight of 168 lbs.)

If this coach then begins to take off fat pounds, his actions are saying, "I believe that optimal weight is important and I should therefore try to follow a sound weight control program." If, on the other hand,

Table 11.2

Skinfolds for Adults—17 Years and Above

Skinfolds (mm)	Males (age in years)				Females (age in years)			
	17-29	30-39	40-49	50 +	16-29	30-39	40-49	50 +
15	4.8	—	—	—	10.5	—	—	—
20	8.1	12.2	12.2	12.6	14.1	17.0	19.8	21.4
25	10.5	14.2	15.0	15.6	16.8	19.4	22.2	24.0
30	12.9	16.2	17.7	18.6	19.5	21.8	24.5	26.6
35	14.7	17.7	19.6	20.8	21.5	23.7	26.4	28.5
40	16.4	19.2	21.4	22.9	23.4	25.5	28.2	30.3
45	17.7	20.4	23.0	24.7	25.0	26.9	29.6	31.9
50	19.0	21.5	24.6	26.5	26.5	28.2	31.0	33.4
55	20.1	22.5	25.9	27.9	27.8	29.4	32.1	34.6
60	21.2	23.5	27.1	29.2	29.1	30.6	33.2	35.7
65	22.2	24.3	28.2	30.4	30.2	31.6	34.1	36.7
70	23.1	25.1	29.3	31.6	31.2	32.5	35.0	37.7
75	24.0	25.9	30.3	32.7	32.2	33.4	35.9	38.7
80	24.8	26.6	31.2	33.8	33.1	34.3	36.7	39.6
85	25.5	27.2	32.1	34.8	34.0	35.1	37.5	40.4
90	26.2	27.8	33.0	35.8	34.8	35.8	38.3	41.2
95	26.9	28.4	33.7	36.6	35.6	36.5	39.0	41.9
100	27.6	29.0	34.4	37.4	36.4	37.2	39.7	42.6
105	28.2	29.6	35.1	38.2	37.1	37.9	40.4	43.3
110	28.8	30.1	35.8	39.0	37.8	38.6	41.0	43.9
115	29.4	30.6	36.4	39.7	38.4	39.1	41.5	44.5
120	30.0	31.1	37.0	40.4	39.0	39.6	42.0	45.1
125	30.5	31.5	37.6	41.1	39.6	40.1	42.5	45.7
130	31.0	31.9	38.2	41.8	40.2	40.6	43.0	46.2
135	31.5	32.3	38.7	42.4	40.8	41.1	43.5	46.7
140	32.0	32.7	39.2	43.0	41.3	41.6	44.0	47.2
145	32.5	33.1	39.7	43.6	41.8	42.1	44.5	47.7
150	32.9	33.5	40.2	44.1	42.3	42.6	45.0	48.2
155	33.3	33.9	40.7	44.6	42.8	43.1	45.4	48.7
160	33.7	34.3	41.2	45.1	43.3	43.6	45.8	49.2
165	34.1	34.6	41.6	45.6	43.7	44.0	46.2	49.6
170	34.5	34.8	42.0	46.1	44.1	44.4	46.6	50.0
175	34.9	—	—	—	—	44.8	47.0	50.4
180	35.3	—	—	—	—	45.2	47.4	50.8
185	35.6	—	—	—	—	45.6	47.8	51.2
190	35.9	—	—	—	—	45.9	48.2	51.6
195	—	—	—	—	—	46.2	48.5	52.0
200	—	—	—	—	—	46.5	48.8	52.4
205	—	—	—	—	—	—	49.1	52.7
210	—	—	—	—	—	—	49.4	53.0

Determination of percent body fat for the sum of the biceps, triceps, subscapula, and iliac skinfolds of males and females 17 years of age and above.

From "Body Fat Assessed from Total Body Density and its Estimation from Skinfold Thickness" by J.V.G.A. Durnin and J. Womersley, *British Journal of Nutrition*, 1974, **32**, 95. Copyright 1974 by the British Journal of Nutrition. Reprinted with permission.

Table 11.3

Calculation of Ideal Weight

Skinfold Total = _100 mm_   Age _30 years_

Sex _Male_   Ideal Percent Fat _16%_

Predicted Percent Fat _29%_

1. Lean Body Weight = Body Weight − (% Fat × Body Weight)

    LBW = 200 lbs − (.29 × 200 lbs)

    142 lbs = 200 lbs − (58 lbs)

2. Ideal Weight = $\dfrac{\text{Lean Body Weight}}{(100\% - \text{Ideal \% Fat})}$

    Ideal Weight = $\dfrac{142 \text{ lbs}}{(1.00 - .16)}$

    168 lbs = $\dfrac{142 \text{ lbs}}{.84}$

---

he takes no actions to reduce his fat weight, there is no reason for his athletes to believe that optimal weight control is important for performance or health reasons.

Furthermore, coaches who are continually seen with a can of pop in one hand and a candy bar in the other will have great difficulty in convincing their athletes of the merits of avoiding junk foods and focusing on complex carbohydrates. Similarly, coaches who skip breakfast and lunch will have a depressed blood glucose level and will likely find themselves in a foul mood by the time practice rolls around. How can such coaches be sensitive to the individual needs of athletes and concentrate on running an efficient and productive practice session?

Weight control is important for effective and efficient performance, and it is true that lean individuals have fewer health problems than do obese individuals. So, preach nutrition and weight control—and practice what you preach!

Appendix A

Body Composition Prediction for Football Players (High School and College-age Males)

The Kelly and Wickkister Equation for Predicting the Ideal Weight of High School and College-age Football Players

The Kelly-Wickkister formula for predicting ideal weight may be used once the following three required measurements have been taken:

Waist Girth

While the athlete is standing, place a metal tape measure (in cm) around the waist in the horizontal plane at the level of the umbilicus.

Triceps Skinfold

Have the athlete stand with the relaxed right arm extended at his or her side. Place the caliper on the vertical fold of skin located midway between the acromion and olecranon processes (shoulder and elbow) as shown in Figure 2.5. (For a more detailed description of skinfold measurement technique, see chapter 2.)

Standing Height

Make the reading (in cm) just after a full inspiration while the athlete is standing with the feet together and heels on the floor.

Record the values from the preceding measurements in the "Actual Measurement" column shown on the right side of Table A-1. To fill in the "Conversion Factor" column, locate the actual measurement value shown on the left side of Table A-1. The conversion factor will be directly to the right. For example, John Smith (see Table A-2) has a waist girth of 80 cm. The conversion factor directly to the right of 80 cm is 38.75. Record this number in the "Conversion Factor" column.

Repeat this same procedure for the triceps skinfold and height measurements. You are now ready to calculate percent fat. To do this, place the waist conversion factor on the line just beneath the constant 0.18 (see right side of Tables A-1 and A-2), then put the triceps conversion factor on the next blank. Now, total the constant, the weight conversion, and the triceps conversion. From this subtotal, subtract the height conversion factor. The answer will be the predicted percent fat.

Because football has a number of positions with many varying responsibilities, there is some variability in the ideal percent fat values for players. Some suggested ideal percent fat values can be found in Table A-3. By using these and the formula found in the bottom right of the recording form, you can determine the ideal playing weight for each player. For example, because John Smith is a defensive back, his ideal percent fat is about 8%. The calculations, then, predict John's maximum weight to be 193 lbs, which means John has to lose 7 lbs of fat.

Table A-1

Conversion Table for Estimating Percent Fat

Name_____ Date_____ Age_____ Weight_____

| Conversion factors | Estimating % fat |

Conversion factors

Waist		Triceps skinfold		Height	
Mea-sure-ment (cm)	Con-ver-sion factor	Mea-sure-ment (mm)	Con-ver-sion factor	Mea-sure-ment (cm)	Con-ver-sion factor
66	31.97	1	0.46	160	28.76
8	32.94	2	0.92	2	29.12
70	33.91	3	1.37	4	29.48
2	34.88	4	1.83	6	29.84
4	35.85	5	2.29	8	30.20
6	36.85	6	2.75	170	30.55
8	37.78	7	3.20	2	30.91
80	38.75	8	3.66	4	31.27
2	39.72	9	4.12	6	31.63
4	40.69	10	4.58	8	31.99
6	41.66	11	5.03	180	32.35
8	42.63	12	5.49	2	32.71
90	43.59	13	5.95	4	33.07
2	44.57	14	6.41	6	33.43
4	45.54	15	6.86	8	33.79
6	46.50	16	7.32	190	34.15
8	47.47	17	7.78	2	34.51
100	48.44	18	8.24	4	34.87
2	49.41	19	8.69	6	35.23
4	50.38	20	9.15	8	35.59
6	51.35	21	9.61	200	35.95
8	52.32	22	10.07	2	36.31
110	53.29	23	10.52	4	36.67
2	54.25	24	10.98	6	37.02
4	55.22	25	11.44	8	37.38
6	56.19	26	11.90	210	37.74
8	57.16	27	12.35		
120	58.13	28	12.81		
2	59.10	29	13.27		
4	60.07	30	13.73		
6	61.02				
8	62.00				

Estimating % fat

Add the constant, the waist, and the triceps conversion factors together; subtract the height conversion factor from that total to get % fat.

	Actual measurements	Conversion factor
1. Waist girth	_____ *cm* =	_____
2. Triceps skinfold	_____ *mm* =	_____
3. Height	_____ *cm* =	_____

Constant   0.18

+ _____ = Waist con-version factor

+ _____ = Triceps con-version factor

_____ = Subtotal

− _____ = Height con-version factor

_____ = % fat

Estimating maximum ideal weight

$$\text{Max. Ideal Wt.} = \frac{\text{LBW}}{(100\% - \text{ideal percent fat})}$$

Max. Ideal Wt. = _____ = _____ =
$$(100\% - \quad)$$

LBW = Weight − Fat Wt. = _____ − _____ =

Fat Wt. = Weight × % Fat = _____

Data in this table are from J.M. Kelly and J.D. Wickkister, "Ideal Football Weight," *The Physician and Sportsmedicine*, 1975, **3**(2), 38-42. Copyright 1975 by McGraw-Hill, Inc. Reprinted with permission.

Table A-2

Sample of a Conversion Table for Estimating Percent Fat

Name_____ Date_____ Age_____ Weight_____

Conversion factors

Estimating % fat

Conversion: Add the constant, the waist, and the triceps conversion factors together; subtract the height conversion factor from that total to get % fat.

Waist		Triceps skinfold		Height	
Measurement (cm)	Conversion factor	Measurement (mm)	Conversion factor	Measurement (cm)	Conversion factor
66	31.97	1	0.46	160	28.76
8	32.94	2	0.92	2	29.12
70	33.91	3	1.37	4	29.48
2	34.88	4	1.83	6	29.84
4	35.85	5	2.29	8	30.20
6	36.85	6	2.75	170	30.55
8	37.78	7	3.20	2	30.91
80	38.75	8	3.66	4	31.27
2	39.72	9	4.12	6	31.63
4	40.69	10	4.58	8	31.99
6	41.66	11	5.03	180	32.35
8	42.63	12	5.49	2	32.71
90	43.59	13	5.95	4	33.07
2	44.57	14	6.41	6	33.43
4	45.54	15	6.86	8	33.79
6	46.50	16	7.32	190	34.15
8	47.47	17	7.78	2	34.51
100	48.44	18	8.24	4	34.87
2	49.41	19	8.69	6	35.23
4	50.38	20	9.15	8	35.59
6	51.35	21	9.61	200	35.95
8	52.32	22	10.07	2	36.31
110	53.29	23	10.52	4	36.67
2	54.25	24	10.98	6	37.02
4	55.22	25	11.44	8	37.38
6	56.19	26	11.90	210	37.74
8	57.16	27	12.35		
120	58.13	28	12.81		
2	59.10	29	13.27		
4	60.07	30	13.73		
6	61.02				
8	62.00				

Example:

	Actual Measurements	Conversion factors
1. Waist girth	80 cm =	38.75
2. Triceps skinfold	10 mm =	4.58
3. Height	180 cm =	32.35

Calculation:

Add constant	0.18	
waist	38.75	
triceps	4.58	
	43.51	subtotal
Subtract height	32.35	
	11.16	% fat

Estimating maximum ideal weight

Conversion: Fat weight = % fat × total weight
Lean body weight = total weight − fat weight
Maximum ideal weight = lean body weight
                        1.00 − % fat desired

*Example: Fat weight = 11.16% × 200 lb = 22.32 lb
Lean body weight = 200 − 22.32 = 177.68 lb
Maximum ideal weight = $\dfrac{177.68}{1.00 - 0.08}$ = 193 lb

*This offensive or defensive back has about 7 extra pounds of fat.

Data in this table are from J.M. Kelly and J.D. Wickkister, "Ideal Football weight," *The Physician and Sportsmedicine*, 1975, 3(2), 38-42. Copyright 1985 by McGraw-Hill, Inc. Reprinted with permission.

Table A-3

Ideal Percent Fat by Position

Position	Ideal % Fat
Defensive back	8
Offensive back	8
Linebackers	15
Offensive lineman, tight ends	15
Defensive lineman	18

Adapted with permission from J.M. Kelly and J.D. Wickkister, "Ideal Football Weight," *The Physician and Sportsmedicine*, 1975, **3**(12), 38-42. Copyright 1975 by McGraw-Hill, Inc.

Appendix *B*

Predicting Ideal Body Weight for Female College-age Gymnasts

The Sinning Equation for the Prediction of Ideal Body Weight for Female College-age Gymnasts

This equation requires that four measurements be taken, including height, weight, neck circumference, and shoulder circumference. A tape measure, preferably a metal one, should be used to take the circumferences. Take the measurements according to the following directions, remembering that any deviation from these directions will jeopardize the accuracy of the prediction.

Standing Height

Have the gymnast stand "as tall as possible" with the feet together and heels on the floor. The athlete should take a deep breath just before the measurement is taken.

Body Weight

Take this with the gymnast in a swim suit and record it to the nearest quarter of a pound.

Neck Circumference

With the gymnast in a standing position, place the tape around the neck at a level just below the larynx or "Adam's Apple." Make sure that the tape is in the horizontal plane and that it is just tense enough to take the slack out.

Shoulder Circumference

Place the tape in the horizontal plane around the shoulder at the level of the widest portion of the deltoid muscle.

Now you are ready for the calculations. Add the figures in Column 3 of Table B-1. Subtract the constant 87.203 from the total. You now have the individual's present or current lean body weight. Since 5-10% (see Table 2.3) has been identified as the ideal percent body fat for women gymnasts, we will use 10% as the ideal value in our sample. Thus, by dividing .90 into the LBW, the ideal weight is derived.

Table B-1

Sinning Equation For the Prediction of Lean Body Weight And Ideal Body Weight for Women Gymnasts

Name _____ Age _____

Season _____ Weight _____

| | Column 1 | Column 2 | Column 3 |

Height _____ cm × .3973 = _____

Shoulder Circumference _____ cm × .8357 = _____

Total = _____

− 87.203

LBW = _____ kg

× 2.2

LBW = _____ lbs

Ideal Weight = $\dfrac{LBW}{(100\% - 10\%*)}$

Ideal Weight = $\dfrac{\underline{\hspace{2cm}}}{.90}$ =

*Note. 10% is the ideal percent fat for female college gymnasts.

From W.E. Sinning, "Anthropometric estimation of body density, fat, and lean body weight in women gymnasts," *Medicine and Science in Sports*, 1978, **10**, 243. Copyright 1978 by the American College of Sports Medicine. Reprinted with permission.

Appendix C
Information for Purchasing a Caliper

We recommend that you purchase a skinfold caliper from:
Lange Skinfold Calipers (about $150.00)
Cambridge Scientific Industries
101 Virginia Ave.
Cambridge, MD 21613

If you are looking for a less expensive caliper, the following products can be purchased (some accuracy is lost, but the most important variable is your experience and knowledge in finding the skinfold sites and using the caliper).

1. Fat-O-Meter ($9.95 plus $1.00 shipping)
   Health and Education Services
   7N015 York Rd.
   Bensenville, IL 60106

2. Physique Meter Kits ($5.95)
   Dr. H., Co.
   P.O. Box 266
   Chesterfield, MO 63017

Appendix D

Nutritive Values of the Edible Part of Food

MILK, CHEESE, CREAM, IMITATION CREAM; RELATED PRODUCTS

Food, Approximate Measure, and Weight (in Grams)		Water (%)	Food Energy (kcal)	Protein (g)	Fat (g)	Fatty Acids Saturated (total) (g)	Fatty Acids Unsaturated Oleic (g)	Fatty Acids Unsaturated Linoleic (g)	Carbohydrate (g)	Calcium (mg)	Iron (mg)	Vitamin A value (I.U.)	Thiamin (mg)	Riboflavin (mg)	Niacin (mg)	Ascorbic acid (mg)
Milk:																
Fluid:																
Whole, 3.5% fat	1 cup	244	87	160	9	9	5	3	Trace	12	288	0.1	350	0.07	0.41	0.2	2
Nonfat (skim)	1 cup	245	90	90	9	Trace	—	—	—	12	296	.1	10	.09	.44	.2	2
Partly skimmed, 2% nonfat milk solids added	1 cup	246	87	145	10	5	3	2	Trace	15	352	.1	200	.10	.52	.2	2
Canned, concentrated, undiluted:																
Evaporated, unsweetened	1 cup	252	74	345	18	20	11	7	1	24	635	.3	810	.10	.86	.5	3
Condensed, sweetened	1 cup	306	27	980	25	27	15	9	1	166	802	.3	1100	.24	1.16	.6	3
Dry, nonfat instant:																
Low-density (1⅓ cups needed for reconstitution to 1 qt)	1 cup	68	4	245	24	Trace	—	—	—	35	879	.4	20[a]	.24	1.21	.6	5
High-density (7/8 cup needed for reconstitution to 1 qt)	1 cup	104	4	375	37	1	—	—	—	54	1345	.6	30[a]	.36	1.85	.9	7
Buttermilk:																
Fluid, cultured, made from skim milk	1 cup	245	90	90	9	Trace	—	—	—	12	296	.1	10	.10	.44	.2	2
Dried, packaged	1 cup	120	3	465	41	6	3	2	Trace	60	1498	.7	260	.31	2.06	1.1	—
Cheese																
Natural:																
Blue or Roquefort type:																
Ounce	1 oz.	28	40	105	6	9	5	3	Trace	1	89	.1	350	.01	.17	.3	0
Cubic inch	1 cu in	17	40	65	4	5	3	2	Trace	Trace	54	.1	210	.01	.11	.2	0
Camembert, packaged in 4-oz pkg with 3 wedges per pkg	1 wedge	38	52	115	7	9	5	3	Trace	1	40	.2	380	.02	.29	.3	0

[a]Value applies to unfortified product; value for fortified low-density product would be 1500 I.U. and the fortified high-density product would be 2290 I.U.

Data are from the Home and Garden Bulletin No. 72, USDA, Washington, DC. Revised 1971.

MILK, CHEESE, CREAM, IMITATION CREAM: RELATED PRODUCTS—Con.

Food, Approximate Measure, and Weight (in Grams)		Weight (g)	Water (%)	Food Energy (kcal)	Protein (g)	Fat (g)	Saturated (total) (g)	Oleic (g)	Linoleic (g)	Carbohydrate (g)	Calcium (mg)	Iron (mg)	Vitamin A value (I.U.)	Thiamin (mg)	Riboflavin (mg)	Niacin (mg)	Ascorbic acid (mg)
Cheese—Continued																	
Cheddar:																	
Ounce	1 oz	28	37	115	7	9	5	3	Trace	1	213	0.3	370	0.01	0.13	Trace	0
Cubic inch	1 cu in	17	37	70	4	6	3	2	Trace	Trace	129	.2	230	.01	.08	Trace	0
Cottage, large or small curd:																	
Creamed:																	
Package of 12-oz net wt	1 pkg	340	78	360	46	14	8	5	Trace	10	320	1.0	580	.10	.85	.3	0
Cup, curd pressed down	1 cup	245	78	260	33	10	6	3	Trace	7	230	.7	420	.07	.61	.2	0
Uncreamed:																	
Package of 12-oz net wt	1 pkg	340	79	290	58	1	1	Trace	Trace	9	306	1.4	30	.10	.95	.3	0
Cup, curd pressed down	1 cup	200	79	170	34	1	Trace	Trace	Trace	5	180	.8	20	.06	.56	.2	0
Cream:																	
Package of 8-oz net wt	1 pkg	227	51	850	18	86	48	28	3	5	141	.5	3500	.05	.54	.2	0
Package of 3-oz net wt	1 pkg	85	51	320	7	32	18	11	1	2	53	.2	1310	.02	.20	.1	0
Cubic-inch	1 cu in	16	51	60	1	6	3	2	Trace	Trace	10	Trace	250	Trace	.04	Trace	0
Parmesan, grated:																	
Cup, pressed down	1 cup	140	17	655	60	43	24	14	1	5	1893	.7	1760	.03	1.22	.3	0
Tablespoon	1 tbsp	5	17	25	2	2	1	Trace	Trace	Trace	68	Trace	60	Trace	.04	Trace	0
Ounce	1 oz	28	17	130	12	9	5	3	Trace	1	383	.1	360	.01	.25	.1	0
Swiss:																	
Ounce	1 oz	28	39	105	8	8	4	3	Trace	1	262	.3	320	Trace	.11	Trace	0
Cubic inch	1 cu in	15	39	55	4	4	2	1	Trace	Trace	139	.1	170	Trace	.06	Trace	0
Pasteurized processed cheese:																	
American:																	
Ounce	1 oz	28	40	105	7	9	5	3	Trace	1	198	.3	350	.01	.12	Trace	0
Cubic inch	1 cu in	18	40	65	4	5	3	2	Trace	Trace	122	.2	210	Trace	.07	Trace	0

Nutrient columns below (continued from the preceding page): approximate measure, weight (grams), water (%), food energy (calories), protein (g), fat (g), saturated fatty acids (g), unsaturated oleic (g), unsaturated linoleic (g), carbohydrate (g), calcium (mg), iron (mg), vitamin A (IU), thiamin (mg), riboflavin (mg), niacin (mg), ascorbic acid (mg).

Item	Measure	g	Water	Food energy	Protein	Fat	Sat.	Oleic	Linoleic	Carb.	Calcium	Iron	Vit. A	Thiamin	Riboflavin	Niacin	Ascorbic acid
Swiss:																	
Ounce	1 oz	28	40	100	8	8	4	3	Trace	1	251	.3	310	Trace	.11	Trace	0
Cubic inch	1 cu in	18	40	65	5	5	3	2	Trace	Trace	159	.2	200	Trace	.07	Trace	0
Pasteurized process cheese food: American:																	
Tablespoon	1 tbsp	14	43	45	3	3	2	1	Trace	1	80	.1	140	Trace	.08	Trace	0
Cubic inch	1 cu in	18	43	60	4	4	2	1	Trace	1	100	.1	170	Trace	.10	Trace	0
Pasteurized process cheese spread, American	1 oz	28	49	80	5	6	3	2	Trace	2	160	.2	250	Trace	.15	Trace	0
Cream:																	
Half-and-half (cream and milk)	1 cup	242	80	325	8	28	15	9	1	11	261	.1	1160	.07	.39	.1	2
Half-and-half (cream and milk)	1 tbsp	15	80	20	1	2	1	1	Trace	1	16	Trace	70	Trace	.02	Trace	Trace
Light, coffee or table	1 cup	240	72	505	7	49	27	16	1	10	245	.1	2020	.07	.36	.1	2
Light, coffee or table	1 tbsp	15	72	30	Trace	3	2	1	Trace	1	15	Trace	130	Trace	.02	Trace	Trace
Sour	1 cup	230	72	485	7	47	26	16	1	10	235	.1	1930	.07	.35	.1	2
Sour	1 tbsp	12	72	25	Trace	2	1	1	Trace	1	12	Trace	100	Trace	.02	Trace	Trace
Whipped topping (pressurized)	1 cup	60	62	155	2	14	8	5	Trace	5	67	Trace	570	Trace	.04	Trace	—
Whipped topping (pressurized)	1 tbsp	3	62	10	Trace	1	Trace	Trace	Trace	Trace	3	—	30	—	Trace	Trace	—
Whipping, unwhipped (volume about double when whipped):																	
Light	1 cup	239	62	715	6	75	41	25	2	7	203	.1	3060	.05	.29	.1	2
Light	1 tbsp	15	62	45	Trace	5	3	2	Trace	Trace	13	Trace	190	Trace	.02	Trace	Trace
Heavy	1 cup	238	57	840	5	90	50	30	3	7	179	.1	3670	.05	.26	.1	2
Heavy	1 tbsp	15	57	55	Trace	6	3	2	Trace	Trace	11	Trace	230	Trace	.02	Trace	Trace
Imitation cream products (made with vegetable fat): Creamers:																	
Powdered	1 cup	94	2	505	4	33	31	1	0	52	21	.6	200[b]	—	Trace	Trace	—
Powdered	1 tsp	2	2	10	Trace	1	Trace	Trace	0	1	1	Trace	Trace[b]	—	—	—	—
Liquid (frozen)	1 cup	245	77	345	2	27	25	0	0	25	29	—	100[b]	0	0	0	—
Liquid (frozen)	1 tbsp	15	77	20	Trace	2	1	0	0	2	2	—	10[b]	0	0	0	—

[b]Contributed largely from beta-carotene used for coloring.

MILK, CHEESE, CREAM, IMITATION CREAM; RELATED PRODUCTS—Con.

Food, Approximate Measure, and Weight (in Grams)		Water (%)	Food Energy (kcal)	Protein (g)	Fat (g)	Fatty Acids Saturated (total) (g)	Unsaturated Oleic (g)	Unsaturated Linoleic (g)	Carbohydrate (g)	Calcium (mg)	Iron (mg)	Vitamin A value (I.U.)	Thiamin (mg)	Riboflavin (mg)	Niacin (mg)	Ascorbic acid (mg)
Imitation cream products (made with vegetable fat):—Con.																
Sour dressing (imitation sour cream) made with nonfat dry milk 1 cup	235	72	440	9	38	35	1	Trace	17	277	.1	10	.07	.38	.2	1
1 tbsp	12	72	20	Trace	2	2	Trace	Trace	1	14	Trace	Trace	Trace	Trace	Trace	Trace
Whipped topping:																
Pressurized 1 cup	70	61	190	1	17	15	1	0	9	5	—	340[b]	—	0	—	—
1 tbsp	4	61	10	Trace	1	1	Trace	0	Trace	Trace	—	20[b]	—	0	—	—
Frozen 1 cup	75	52	230	1	20	18	Trace	0	15	5	—	560[b]	—	0	—	—
1 tbsp	4	52	10	Trace	1	1	Trace	0	1	Trace	—	30[b]	—	0	—	—
Powdered, made with whole milk 1 cup	75	58	175	3	12	10	1	Trace	15	62	Trace	330[b]	.02	.08	.1	Trace
1 tbsp	4	58	10	Trace	1	1	Trace	Trace	1	3	Trace	20	Trace	Trace	Trace	Trace
Milk beverages:																
Cocoa, homemade 1 cup	250	79	245	10	12	7	4	Trace	27	295	1.0	400	.10	.45	.5	3
Chocolate-flavored drink made with skim milk and 2% added butterfat 1 cup	250	83	190	8	6	3	2	Trace	27	270	.5	210	.10	.40	.3	3
Malted milk:																
Dry powder, approx. 3 heaping teaspoons/oz 1 oz.	28	3	115	4	2	—	—	—	20	82	.6	290	.09	.15	.1	0
Beverage 1 cup	235	78	245	11	10	—	—	—	28	317	.7	590	.14	.49	.2	2
Milk desserts:																
Custard, baked 1 cup	265	77	305	14	15	7	5	1	29	297	1.1	930	.11	.50	.3	1
Ice cream:																
Regular (approx. 10% fat) ½ gal	1064	63	2055	48	113	62	37	3	221	1553	.5	4680	.43	2.23	1.1	11
1 cup	133	63	255	6	14	8	5	Trace	28	194	.1	590	.05	.28	.1	1
3 fl oz	50	63	95	2	5	3	2	Trace	10	73	Trace	220	.02	.11	.1	1
Rich (approx. 16% fat) ½ gal	1188	63	2635	31	191	105	63	6	214	927	.2	7840	.24	1.31	1.2	12
1 cup	148	63	330	4	24	13	8	1	27	115	Trace	980	.03	.16	.1	1

Ice milk:																	
Hardened	½ gal	1048	67	1595	50	53	29	17	2	235	1635	1.0	2200	.52	2.31	1.0	10
	1 cup	131	67	200	6	7	4	2	Trace	29	204	.1	280	.07	.29	.1	1
Soft-serve	1 cup	175	67	265	8	9	5	3	Trace	39	273	.2	370	.09	.39	.2	2
Yogurt																	
Made from partially skimmed milk	1 cup	245	89	125	8	4	2	1	Trace	13	294	.1	170	.10	.44	.2	2
Made from whole milk	1 cup	245	88	150	7	8	5	3	Trace	12	272	.1	340	.07	.39	.2	2

EGGS

Eggs, large, 24 ounces per dozen:

Raw or cooked in shell or with nothing added:

Whole, without shell	1 egg	50	74	80	6	6	2	3	Trace	Trace	27	1.1	590	.05	.15	Trace	0
White of egg	1 white	33	88	15	4	Trace	—	—	—	Trace	3	Trace	0	Trace	.09	Trace	0
Yolk of egg	1 yolk	17	51	60	3	5	2	2	Trace	Trace	24	.9	580	.04	.07	Trace	0
Scrambled with milk and fat	1 egg	64	72	110	7	8	3	3	Trace	1	51	1.1	690	.05	.18	Trace	0

MEAT, POULTRY, FISH, SHELLFISH; RELATED PRODUCTS

Bacon, (20 slices per lb raw) 2 slices broiled or fried, crisp		15	8	90	5	8	3	4	1	1	2	.5	0	.08	.05	.8	—
Beef,[c] cooked:																	
Cuts braised, simmered, or pot roasted:																	
Lean and fat	3 oz	85	53	245	23	16	8	7	Trace	0	10	2.9	30	.04	.18	3.5	—
Lean only	2.5 oz	72	62	140	22	5	2	2	Trace	0	10	2.7	10	.04	.16	3.3	—
Hamburger (ground beef), broiled:																	
Lean	3 oz	85	60	185	23	10	5	4	Trace	0	10	3.0	20	.08	.20	5.1	—
Regular	3 oz	85	54	245	21	17	8	8	Trace	0	9	2.7	30	.07	.18	4.6	—
Roast, overcooked, no liquid added:																	
Relatively fat, such as rib:																	
Lean and fat	3 oz	85	40	375	17	34	16	15	1	0	8	2.2	70	.05	.13	3.1	—
Lean only	1.8 oz	51	57	125	14	7	3	3	Trace	0	6	1.8	10	.04	.11	2.6	—
Relatively lean, such as heel of round:																	
Lean and fat	3 oz	85	62	165	25	7	3	3	Trace	0	11	3.2	10	.06	.19	4.5	—
Lean only	2.7 oz	78	65	125	24	3	1	1	Trace	0	10	3.0	Trace	.06	.18	4.3	—

b Contributed largely from beta-carotene used for coloring.

c Outer layer of fat on the cut was removed to within approximately ½-in. of the lean. Deposits of fat within the cut were not removed.

MEAT, POULTRY, FISH, SHELLFISH; RELATED PRODUCTS—Con.

Food, Approximate Measure, and Weight (in Grams)		Water (%)	Food Energy (kcal)	Protein (g)	Fat (g)	Fatty Acids				Carbohydrate (g)	Calcium (mg)	Iron (mg)	Vitamin A value (I.U.)	Thiamin (mg)	Riboflavin (mg)	Niacin (mg)	Ascorbic acid (mg)
						Saturated (total) (g)	Unsaturated										
							Oleic (g)	Linoleic (g)									
Steak, broiled:																	
Relatively fat, such as sirloin:																	
Lean and fat	3 oz	85	44	330	20	27	13	12	1	0	9	2.5	50	.05	.16	4.0	—
Lean only	2 oz	56	59	115	18	4	2	2	Trace	0	7	2.2	10	.05	.14	3.6	—
Relatively lean, such as round:																	
Lean and fat	3 oz	85	55	220	24	13	6	6	Trace	0	10	3.0	20	.07	.19	4.8	—
Lean only	2.4 oz	68	61	130	21	4	2	2	Trace	0	9	2.5	10	.06	.16	4.1	—
Beef, Canned:																	
Corned beef	3 oz	85	59	185	22	10	5	4	Trace	0	17	3.7	20	.01	.20	2.9	—
Corned beef hash	3 oz	85	67	155	7	10	5	4	Trace	9	11	1.7	—	.01	.08	1.8	—
Beef, dried or chipped	2 oz	57	48	115	19	4	2	2	Trace	0	11	2.9		.04	.18	2.2	—
Beef and vegetable stew	1 cup	235	82	210	15	10	5	4	Trace	15	28	2.8	2310	.13	.17	4.4	15
Beef pot pie, baked	1 pie	227	55	560	23	33	9	20	2	43	32	4.1	1860	.25	.27	4.5	7
4¼-in. diam., weight before baking about 8 oz																	
Chicken, cooked:																	
Flesh only, broiled	3 oz	85	71	115	20	3	1	1	1	0	8	1.4	80	.05	.16	7.4	—
Breast, fried, ½ breast:																	
With bone	3.3 oz	94	58	155	25	5	1	2	1	1	9	1.3	70	.04	.17	11.2	—
Flesh and skin only	2.7 oz	76	58	155	25	5	1	2	1	1	9	1.3	70	.04	.17	11.2	—
Drumstick, fried:																	
With bone	2.1 oz	59	55	90	12	4	1	2	1	Trace	6	.9	50	.03	.15	2.7	—
Flesh and skin only	1.3 oz	38	55	90	12	4	1	2	1	Trace	6	.9	50	.03	.15	2.7	—
Chicken, canned, boneless	3 oz	85	65	170	18	10	3	4	2	0	18	1.3	200	.03	.11	3.7	3
Chicken pot pie, baked	1 pie	227	57	535	23	31	10	15	3	42	68	3.0	3020	.25	.26	4.1	5
4¼-in. diam., weight before baking about 8 oz																	

	Measure	Grams	Water %	Food energy	Protein	Fat	Saturated	Oleic	Linoleic	Carbohydrate	Calcium	Iron	Vitamin A	Thiamin	Riboflavin	Niacin	Ascorbic acid
Chili con carne, canned:																	
With beans	1 cup	250	72	335	19	15	7	7	Trace	30	80	4.2	150	.08	.18	3.2	—
Without beans	1 cup	255	67	510	26	38	18	17	1	15	97	3.6	380	.05	.31	5.6	—
Heart, beef, lean, braised	3 oz	85	61	160	27	5	—	—	—	1	5	5.0	20	.21	1.04	6.5	1
Lamb,[c] cooked																	
Chop, thick, with bone, 1 chop, broiled	4.8 oz	137	47	400	25	33	18	12	1	0	10	1.5	—	.14	.25	5.6	—
Lean and fat	4 oz	112	47	400	25	33	18	12	1	0	10	1.5	—	.14	.25	5.6	—
Lean only	2.6 oz	74	62	140	21	6	3	2	Trace	0	9	1.5	—	.11	.20	4.5	—
Leg roasted:																	
Lean and fat	3 oz	85	54	235	22	16	9	6	Trace	0	9	1.4	—	.13	.23	4.7	—
Lean only	2.5 oz	71	62	130	20	5	3	2	Trace	0	9	1.4	—	.12	.21	4.4	—
Shoulder, roasted:																	
Lean and fat	3 oz	85	50	285	18	23	13	8	1	0	9	1.0	—	.11	.20	4.0	—
Lean only	2.3 oz	64	61	130	17	6	3	2	Trace	0	8	1.0	—	.10	.18	3.7	—
Liver, beef, fried	2 oz	57	57	130	15	6	—	—	—	3	6	5.0	30,280	.15	2.37	9.4	15
Pork, cured, cooked:																	
Ham, light cure, lean and fat, roasted	3 oz	85	54	245	18	19	7	8	2	0	8	2.2	0	.40	.16	3.1	—
Luncheon meat:																	
Boiled ham, sliced	2 oz	57	59	135	11	10	4	4	1	0	6	1.6	0	.25	.09	1.5	—
Canned, spiced or unspiced	2 oz	57	55	165	8	14	5	6	1	1	5	1.2	0	.18	.12	1.6	—
Pork, fresh,[c] cooked:																	
Chop, thick, with bone	3.5 oz	98	42	260	16	21	8	9	2	0	8	2.2	0	.63	.18	3.8	—
Lean and fat	2.3 oz	66	42	260	16	21	8	9	2	0	8	2.2	0	.63	.18	3.8	—
Lean only	1.7 oz	48	53	130	15	7	2	3	1	0	7	1.9	0	.54	.16	3.3	—
Roast, oven-cooked, no liquid added:																	
Lean and fat	3 oz	85	46	310	21	24	9	10	2	0	9	2.7	0	.78	.22	4.7	—
Lean only	2.4 oz	68	55	175	20	10	4	4	1	0	9	2.6	0	.73	.21	4.4	—
Cuts, simmered:																	
Lean and fat	3 oz	85	46	320	20	26	9	11	2	0	8	2.5	0	.46	.21	4.1	—
Lean only	2.2 oz	63	60	135	18	6	2	3	1	0	8	2.3	0	.42	.19	3.7	—
Sausage:																	
Bologna, slice, 3-in. diam. by 1/8 in.	2 slices	26	56	80	3	7	—	—	—	Trace	2	.5	—	.04	.06	.7	—

[c]Outer layer of fat on the cut was removed to within approximately ½-in. of the lean. Deposits of fat within the cut were not removed.

MEAT, POULTRY, FISH, SHELLFISH; RELATED PRODUCTS—Con.

Food, Approximate Measure, and Weight (in Grams)			Water (%)	Food Energy (kcal)	Protein (g)	Fat (g)	Fatty Acids Saturated (total) (g)	Unsaturated Oleic (g)	Linoleic (g)	Carbohydrate (g)	Calcium (mg)	Iron (mg)	Vitamin A value (I.U.)	Thiamin (mg)	Riboflavin (mg)	Niacin (mg)	Ascorbic acid (mg)
Sausage:—Con.																	
Braunschweiger, slice 2-in. diam. by ¼ in.	2 slices	20	53	65	3	5	—	—	—	Trace	2	1.2	1310	.03	.29	1.6	—
Deviled ham, canned	1 tbsp	13	51	45	2	4	2	2	Trace	0	1	.3	—	.02	.01	.2	—
Frankfurter, heated (8 per lb. purchased pkg)	1 frank	56	57	170	7	15	—	—	—	1	3	.8	—	.08	.11	1.4	—
Pork links, cooked (16 links per lb. raw)	2 links	26	35	125	5	11	4	5	1	Trace	2	.6	0	.21	.09	1.0	—
Salami, dry type	1 oz	28	30	130	7	11	—	—	—	Trace	4	1.0	—	.10	.07	1.5	—
Salami, cooked	1 oz	28	51	90	5	7	—	—	—	Trace	3	.7	—	.07	.07	1.2	—
Vienna, canned (7 sausages per 5-oz can)	1 sausage	16	63	40	2	3	—	—	—	Trace	1	.3	—	.01	.02	.4	—
Veal, medium fat, cooked, bone removed:																	
Cutlet	3 oz	85	60	185	23	9	5	4	Trace	—	9	2.7	—	.06	.21	4.6	—
Roast	3 oz	85	55	230	23	14	7	6	Trace	0	10	2.9	—	.11	.26	6.6	—
Fish and shellfish:																	
Bluefish, baked with table fat	3 oz	85	68	135	22	4	—	—	—	0	25	.6	40	.09	.08	1.6	—
Clams:																	
Raw, meat only	3 oz	85	82	65	11	1	—	—	—	2	59	5.2	90	.08	.15	1.1	8
Canned, solids and liquid	3 oz	85	86	45	7	1	—	—	—	2	47	3.5	—	.01	.09	.9	—
Crabmeat, canned	3 oz	85	77	85	15	2	—	—	—	1	38	.7	—	.07	.07	1.6	—
Fish sticks, breaded, cooked, frozen; stick 3¾ by 1 by ½ in	10 sticks or 8 oz pkg	227	66	400	38	20	5	4	10	15	25	0.9	—	.09	.16	3.6	—
Haddock, breaded, fried	3 oz	85	66	140	17	5	1	3	Trace	5	34	1.0	—	.03	.06	2.7	2
Ocean perch, breaded, fried	3 oz	85	59	195	16	11	—	—	—	6	28	1.1	—	.08	.09	1.5	—
Oysters, raw, meat only (13-19 med. selects)	1 cup	240	85	160	20	4	—	—	—	8	226	13.2	740	.33	.43	6.0	—

Salmon, pink, canned	3 oz	85	71	120	17	5	1	1	1	0	167[d]	.7	60	.03	.16	6.8	—
Sardines, Atlantic, canned in oil, drained solid	3 oz	85	62	175	20	9	—	—	Trace	0	372	2.5	190	.02	.17	4.6	—
Shad, baked with table fat and bacon	3 oz	85	64	170	20	10	—	—	—	0	20	.5	20	.11	.22	7.3	—
Shrimp, canned, meat	3 oz	85	70	100	21	1	—	—	—	1	98	2.6	50	.01	.03	1.5	—
Swordfish, broiled with butter or margarine	3 oz	85	65	150	24	5	—	—	—	0	23	1.1	1750	.03	.04	9.3	—
Tuna, canned in oil, drained solids	3 oz	85	61	170	24	7	2	1	1	0	7	1.6	70	.04	.10	10.1	—

MATURE DRY BEANS AND PEAS, NUTS, PEANUTS; RELATED PRODUCTS

Almonds, Shelled whole kernels	1 cup	142	5	850	26	77	6	52	15	28	332	6.7	0	.34	1.31	5.0	Trace
Beans, dry:																	
Common varieties as Great Northern, navy, and others:																	
Cooked, drained:																	
Great Northern	1 cup	180	69	210	14	1	—	—	—	38	90	4.9	0	.25	.13	1.3	0
Navy (pea)	1 cup	190	69	225	15	1	—	—	—	40	95	5.1	0	.27	.13	1.3	0
Canned, solids and liquid:																	
White with —																	
Frankfurters (sliced)	1 cup	255	71	365	19	18	—	—	—	32	94	4.8	330	.18	.15	3.3	Trace
Pork and tomato sauce	1 cup	255	71	310	16	7	2	3	1	49	138	4.6	330	.20	.08	1.5	5
Pork and sweet sauce	1 cup	255	66	385	16	12	4	5	1	54	161	5.9	—	.15	.10	1.3	—
Red kidney	1 cup	255	76	230	15	1	—	—	—	42	74	4.6	10	.13	.10	1.5	—
Lima, cooked, drained	1 cup	190	64	260	16	1	—	—	—	49	55	5.9	—	.25	.11	1.3	—
Cashew nuts, roasted	1 cup	140	5	785	24	64	11	45	4	41	53	5.3	140	.60	.35	2.5	—
Coconut, fresh, meat only:																	
Pieces, approx. 2 by 2 by 1/2 in	1 piece	45	51	155	2	16	14	1	Trace	4	6	.8	0	.02	.01	.2	1
Shredded or grated, firmly packed	1 cup	130	51	450	5	46	39	3	Trace	12	17	2.2	0	.07	.03	.7	4
Cowpeas or blackeye peas, dry, cooked	1 cup	248	80	190	13	1	—	—	—	34	42	3.2	20	.41	.11	1.1	Trace
Peanuts, roasted, salted, halves	1 cup	144	2	840	37	72	16	31	21	27	107	3.0	—	.46	.19	24.7	0

[d] If bones are discarded, value will be greatly reduced.

Food, Approximate Measure, and Weight (in Grams)		Water (%)	Food Energy (kcal)	Protein (g)	Fat (g)	Fatty Acids Saturated (total) (g)	Unsaturated Oleic (g)	Linoleic (g)	Carbohydrate (g)	Calcium (mg)	Iron (mg)	Vitamin A value (I.U.)	Thiamin (mg)	Riboflavin (mg)	Niacin (mg)	Ascorbic acid (mg)
MATURE DRY BEANS AND PEAS, NUTS, PEANUTS; RELATED PRODUCTS—Con.																
Peanut butter	1 tbsp	16	2	95	4	8	2	4	2	3	9	.3	—	.02	.02	2.4	0
Peas, split, dry, cooked	1 cup	250	70	290	20	1	—	—	—	52	28	4.2	100	.37	.22	2.2	—
Pecans, halves	1 cup	108	3	740	10	77	5	48	15	16	79	2.6	140	.93	.14	1.0	2
Walnuts, black or native	1 cup	126	3	790	26	75	4	26	36	19	Trace	7.6	380	.28	.14	.9	—
VEGETABLES AND VEGETABLE PRODUCTS																
Asparagus, green:																	
Cooked, drained:																	
Spears, ½-in diam. at base	4 spears	60	94	10	1	Trace	—	—	—	2	13	.4	540	.10	.11	.8	16
Pieces, 1½ - 2-in lengths	1 cup	145	94	30	3	Trace	—	—	—	5	30	.9	1310	.23	.26	2.0	38
Canned, solids and liquid	1 cup	244	94	45	5	1	—	—	—	7	44	4.1	1240	.15	.22	2.0	37
Beans:																	
Lima, immature seeds, cooked, drained	1 cup	170	71	190	13	1	—	—	—	34	80	4.3	480	.31	.17	2.2	29
Snap:																	
Green:																	
Cooked, drained	1 cup	125	92	30	2	Trace	—	—	—	7	63	.8	680	.09	.11	.6	15
Canned, solids and liquid	1 cup	239	94	45	2	Trace	—	—	—	10	81	2.9	690	.07	.10	.7	10
Yellow or Wax:																	
Cooked, drained	1 cup	125	93	30	2	Trace	—	—	—	6	63	0.8	290	.09	.11	.6	16
Canned, solids and liquid	1 cup	239	94	45	2	1	—	—	—	10	81	2.9	140	.07	.10	.7	12
Sprouted mung beans, cooked, drained	1 cup	125	91	35	4	Trace	—	—	—	7	21	1.1	30	.11	.13	.9	8

Food	Measure																
Beets																	
Cooked, drained, peeled:																	
Whole beets, 2-in diam.	2 beets	100	91	30	1	Trace	—	—	—	7	14	.5	20	.03	.04	.3	6
Diced or sliced	1 cup	170	91	55	2	Trace	—	—	—	12	24	.9	30	.05	.07	.5	10
Canned, solids and liquid	1 cup	246	90	85	2	Trace	—	—	—	19	34	1.5	20	.02	.05	.2	7
Beet greens, leaves and stems, cooked, drained	1 cup	145	94	25	3	Trace	—	—	—	5	144	2.8	7,400	.10	.22	.4	22
Blackeye peas. See Cowpeas.																	
Broccoli, cooked, drained:																	
Whole stalks, medium size	1 stalk	180	91	45	6	1	—	—	—	8	158	1.4	4,500	.16	.36	1.4	162
Stalks cut into ½-in pieces	1 cup	155	91	40	5	1	—	—	—	7	136	1.2	3,880	.14	.31	1.2	140
Chopped, yield from 10-oz frozen pkg	1-3/8 cups	250	92	65	7	1	—	—	—	12	135	1.8	6,500	.15	.30	1.3	143
Brussels sprouts, 7-8 sprouts (1¼ - 1½-in diam) per cup, cooked	1 cup	155	88	55	7	1	—	—	—	10	50	1.7	810	.12	.22	1.2	135
Cabbage:																	
Common varieties:																	
Raw:																	
Coarsely shredded or sliced	1 cup	70	92	15	1	Trace	—	—	—	4	34	.3	90	.04	.04	.2	33
Finely shredded or chopped	1 cup	90	92	20	1	Trace	—	—	—	5	44	.4	120	.05	.05	.3	42
Cooked	1 cup	145	94	30	2	Trace	—	—	—	6	64	.4	190	.06	.06	.4	48
Red, raw, coarsely shredded	1 cup	70	90	20	1	Trace	—	—	—	5	29	.6	30	.06	.04	.3	43
Savoy, raw, coarsely shredded	1 cup	70	92	15	2	Trace	—	—	—	3	47	.6	140	.04	.06	.2	39
Cabbage, celery or Chinese, raw, cut in 1-in pieces	1 cup	75	95	10	1	Trace	—	—	—	2	32	.5	110	.04	.03	.5	19
Cabbage, spoon (or pakchoy), cooked	1 cup	170	95	25	2	Trace	—	—	—	4	252	1.0	5,270	.07	.14	1.2	26
Carrots:																	
Raw:																	
Whole, 5½ by 1 in (25 thin strips)	1 carrot	50	88	20	1	Trace	—	—	—	5	18	.4	5,500	.03	.03	.3	4
Grated	1 cup	110	88	45	1	Trace	—	—	—	11	41	.8	12,100	.06	.06	.7	9

Food, Approximate Measure, and Weight (in Grams)			Water (%)	Food Energy (kcal)	Protein (g)	Fat (g)	Fatty Acids Saturated (total) (g)	Unsaturated Oleic (g)	Linoleic (g)	Carbohydrate (g)	Calcium (mg)	Iron (mg)	Vitamin A value (I.U.)	Thiamin (mg)	Riboflavin (mg)	Niacin (mg)	Ascorbic acid (mg)
VEGETABLES AND VEGETABLE PRODUCTS—Con.																	
Cooked, diced	1 cup	145	91	45	1	Trace	—	—	—	10	48	.9	15,220	.08	.07	.7	9
Canned, strained or chopped (baby food)	1 oz	28	92	10	Trace	Trace	—	—	—	2	7	.1	3,690	.01	.01	.1	1
Cauliflower, cooked, flowerbuds	1 cup	120	93	25	3	Trace	—	—	—	5	25	.8	70	.11	.10	.7	66
Celery, raw:																	
Stalk, large outer, 8 by about 1½ in, at root end	1 stalk	40	94	5	Trace	Trace	—	—	—	2	16	.1	100	.01	.01	.1	4
Pieces, diced	1 cup	100	94	15	1	Trace	—	—	—	4	39	.3	240	.03	.03	.3	0
Collards, cooked	1 cup	190	91	55	5	1	—	—	—	9	289	1.1	10,260	.27	.37	2.4	87
Corn, sweet:																	
Cooked, ear 5 by 1¾ in[e]	1 ear	140	74	70	3	1	—	—	—	16	2	.5	310[f]	.09	.08	1.0	7
Canned, solids and liquid	1 cup	256	81	170	5	2	—	—	—	40	10	1.0	690[f]	.07	.12	2.3	13
Cowpeas, cooked, immature seeds	1 cup	160	72	175	13	1	—	—	—	29	38	3.4	560	.49	.18	2.3	28
Cucumbers, 10 oz; 7½ by about 2 in:																	
Raw, pared	1 cucumber	207	96	30	1	Trace	—	—	—	7	35	.6	Trace	.07	.09	.4	23
Raw, pared, center slice 1/8-in thick	6 slices	50	96	5	Trace	Trace	—	—	—	2	8	.2	Trace	.02	.02	.1	6
Dandelion greens, cooked	1 cup	180	90	60	4	1	—	—	—	12	252	3.2	21,060	.24	.29	—	32
Endive, curly (including escarole)	2 oz	57	93	10	1	Trace	—	—	—	2	46	1.0	1,870	.04	.08	.3	6
Kale, leaves including stems, cooked	1 cup	110	91	30	4	1	—	—	—	4	147	1.3	8,140	—	—	—	68
Lettuce, raw:																	
Butterhead, as Boston types; head, 4-in diam.	1 head	220	95	30	3	Trace	—	—	—	6	77	4.4	2,130	.14	.13	.6	18
Crisphead, as Iceberg; head, 4¾-in diam.	1 head	454	96	60	4	Trace	—	—	—	13	91	2.3	1,500	.29	.27	1.3	29

Food	Measure																	
Looseleaf, or bunching varieties, leaves	2 large	50	94	10	1	Trace	—	—	—	2	34	.7	950	.03	.04	.2	9
Mushrooms, canned, solids and liquid	1 cup	244	93	40	5	Trace	—	—	—	6	15	1.2	Trace	.04	.60	4.8	4
Mustard greens, cooked	1 cup	140	93	35	3	1	—	—	—	6	193	2.5	8,120	.11	.19	.9	68
Okra, cooked, pod, 3 by 5/8 in	8 pods	85	91	25	2	Trace	—	—	—	5	78	.4	420	.11	.15	.8	17
Onions: Mature: Raw, onion 2½-in diam.	1 onion	110	89	40	2	Trace	—	—	—	10	30	.6	40	.04	.04	.2	11
Cooked	1 cup	210	92	60	3	Trace	—	—	—	14	50	.8	80	.06	.06	.4	14
Young green, small, without tops	6 onions	50	88	20	1	Trace	—	—	—	5	20	.3	Trace	.02	.02	.2	12
Parsley, raw, chopped	1 tbsp	4	85	Trace	Trace	Trace	—	—	—	Trace	8	.2	340	Trace	.01	Trace	7
Parsnips, cooked	1 cup	155	82	100	2	1	—	—	—	23	70	.9	50	.11	.12	.2	16
Peas, green: Cooked	1 cup	160	82	115	9	1	—	—	—	19	37	2.9	860	.44	.17	3.7	33
Canned, solids and liquid	1 cup	249	83	165	9	1	—	—	—	31	50	4.2	1,120	.23	.13	2.2	22
Canned, strained (baby food)	1 oz	28	86	15	1	Trace	—	—	—	3	3	.4	140	.02	.02	.4	3
Peppers, hot, red, without seeds, dried (ground chili powder), added seasonings	1 tbsp	15	8	50	2	2	—	—	—	8	40	2.3	9,750	.03	.17	1.3	2
Peppers, sweet: Raw, about 5 per pound: Green pod without stem and seeds	1 pod	74	93	15	1	Trace	—	—	—	4	7	.5	310	.06	.06	.4	94
Cooked, boiled, drained	1 pod	73	95	15	1	Trace	—	—	—	3	7	.4	310	.05	.05	.4	70
Potatoes, medium (about 3 per pound raw): Baked, peeled after baking	1 potato	99	75	90	3	Trace	—	—	—	21	9	.7	Trace	.10	.04	1.7	20
Boiled: Peeled after boiling	1 potato	136	80	105	3	Trace	—	—	—	23	10	.8	Trace	.13	.05	2.0	22
Peeled before boiling	1 potato	122	83	80	2	Trace	—	—	—	18	7	.6	Trace	.11	.04	1.4	20

[e] Measure and weight apply to entire vegetable or fruit including parts not usually eaten.

[f] Based on yellow varieties; white varieties contain only a trace of cryptoxanthin and carotenes, the pigments in corn that have biological activity.

Food, Approximate Measure, and Weight (in Grams)		Weight (g)	Water (%)	Food Energy (kcal)	Protein (g)	Fat (g)	Fatty Acids Saturated (total) (g)	Unsaturated Oleic (g)	Lin- oleic (g)	Carbo- hy- drate (g)	Cal- cium (mg)	Iron (mg)	Vita- min A value (I.U.)	Thia- min (mg)	Ribo- flavin (mg)	Niacin (mg)	Ascor- bic acid (mg)
VEGETABLES AND VEGETABLE PRODUCTS—Con.																	
Potatoes—Con.																	
French-fried, piece 2 by ½ by ½ in:																	
Cooked in deep fat	10 pieces	57	45	155	2	7	2	2	4	20	9	.7	Trace	.07	.04	1.8	12
Frozen, heated	10 pieces	57	53	125	2	5	1	1	2	19	5	1.0	Trace	.08	.01	1.5	12
Mashed:																	
Milk added	1 cup	195	83	125	4	1	—	—	—	25	47	.8	50	.16	.10	2.0	19
Milk and butter added	1 cup	195	80	185	4	8	4	3	Trace	24	47	.8	330	.16	.10	1.9	18
Potato chips, medium, 2-in diam.	10 chips	20	2	115	1	8	2	2	4	10	8	.4	Trace	.04	.01	1.0	3
Pumpkin, canned	1 cup	228	90	75	2	1	—	—	—	18	57	.9	14,590	.07	.12	1.3	12
Radishes, raw, small, without tops	4 radishes	40	94	5	Trace	Trace	—	—	—	1	12	.4	Trace	.01	.01	.1	10
Sauerkraut, canned, solids and liquid	1 cup	235	93	45	2	Trace	—	—	—	9	85	1.2	120	.07	.09	.4	33
Spinach:																	
Cooked	1 cup	180	92	40	5	1	—	—	—	6	167	4.0	14,580	.13	.25	1.0	50
Canned, drained solids	1 cup	180	91	45	5	1	—	—	—	6	212	4.7	14,400	.03	.21	.6	24
Squash:																	
Cooked:																	
Summer, diced	1 cup	210	96	30	2	Trace	—	—	—	7	52	.8	820	.10	.16	1.6	21
Winter, baked, mashed	1 cup	205	81	130	4	1	—	—	—	32	57	1.6	8,610	.10	.27	1.4	27
Sweet potatoes:																	
Cooked, medium, 5 by 2 in, weight raw about 6 oz																	
Baked, peeled after baking	1 sweet- potato	110	64	155	2	1	—	—	—	36	44	1.0	8,910	.10	.07	.7	24
Boiled, peeled after boiling	1 sweet- potato	147	71	170	2	1	—	—	—	39	47	1.0	11,610	.13	.09	.9	25
Candied, 3½ by 2¼-in	1 sweet- potato	175	60	295	2	6	2	3	1	60	65	1.6	11,030	.10	.08	.8	17

Food	Measure	Grams	Water (%)	Food energy (calories)	Protein (g)	Fat (g)	Saturated fatty acids (g)	Oleic (g)	Linoleic (g)	Carbohydrate (g)	Calcium (mg)	Iron (mg)	Vitamin A (IU)	Thiamine (mg)	Riboflavin (mg)	Niacin (mg)	Ascorbic acid (mg)
Canned, vacuum or solid pack	1 cup	218	72	235	4	Trace	—	—	—	54	54	1.7	17,000	.10	.10	1.4	30
Tomatoes:																	
Raw, approx. 3-in diam. 2-1/8-in high; wt 7 oz	1 tomato	200	90	40	2	Trace	—	—	—	9	24	.9	1,640	.11	.07	1.3	42[g]
Canned, solids and liquid	1 cup	241	94	50	2	1	—	—	—	10	14	1.2	2,170	.12	.07	1.7	41
Tomato catsup:																	
Cup	1 cup	273	69	290	6	1	—	—	—	69	60	2.2	3,820	.25	.19	4.4	41
Tablespoon	1 tbsp	15	69	15	Trace	Trace	—	—	—	4	3	.1	210	.01	.01	.2	2
Tomato juice, canned:																	
Cup	1 cup	243	94	45	2	Trace	—	—	—	10	17	2.2	1,940	.12	.07	1.9	39
Glass (6 fl oz)	1 glass	182	94	35	2	Trace	—	—	—	8	13	1.6	1,460	.09	.05	1.5	29
Turnips, cooked, diced	1 cup	155	94	35	1	Trace	—	—	—	8	54	.6	Trace	.06	.08	.5	34
Turnip greens, cooked	1 cup	145	94	30	3	Trace	—	—	—	5	252	1.5	8,270	.15	.33	.7	68
FRUITS AND FRUIT PRODUCTS																	
Apples, raw (about 3 per lb)[e]	1 apple	150	85	70	Trace	Trace	—	—	—	18	8	.4	50	.04	.02	.1	3
Apple juice, bottled or canned	1 cup	248	88	120	Trace	Trace	—	—	—	30	15	1.5	—	.02	.05	.2	2
Applesauce, canned:																	
Sweetened	1 cup	255	76	230	1	Trace	—	—	—	61	10	1.3	100	.05	.03	.1	3[h]
Unsweetened or artificially sweetened	1 cup	244	88	100	1	Trace	—	—	—	26	10	1.2	100	.05	.02	.1	2[h]
Apricots:																	
Raw (about 12 per lb)[e]	3 apricots	114	85	55	1	Trace	—	—	—	14	18	.5	2,890	.03	.04	.7	10
Canned in heavy syrup	1 cup	259	77	220	2	Trace	—	—	—	57	28	.8	4,510	.05	.06	.9	10
Dried, uncooked (40 halves per cup)	1 cup	150	25	390	8	1	—	—	—	100	100	8.2	16,350	.02	.23	4.9	19
Cooked, unsweetened, fruit and liquid	1 cup	285	76	240	5	1	—	—	—	62	63	5.1	8,550	.01	.13	2.8	8
Apricot nectar, canned	1 cup	251	85	140	1	Trace	—	—	—	37	23	.5	2,380	.03	.03	.5	8[h]

[e]Measure and weight apply to entire vegetable or fruit including parts not usually eaten.

[g]Year-round average. Samples marketed from November through May, average 20 milligrams per 200-gram tomato; from June through October, around 52 milligrams.

[h]This is the amount from the fruit. Additional ascorbic acid may be added by the manufacturer. Refer to the label for this information.

FRUITS AND FRUIT PRODUCTS—Con.

Food, Approximate Measure, and Weight (in Grams)			Water (%)	Food Energy (kcal)	Protein (g)	Fat (g)	Fatty Acids Saturated (total) (g)	Unsaturated Oleic (g)	Unsaturated Linoleic (g)	Carbohydrate (g)	Calcium (mg)	Iron (mg)	Vitamin A value (I.U.)	Thiamin (mg)	Riboflavin (mg)	Niacin (mg)	Ascorbic acid (mg)
Avocados, whole fruit, raw[e]																	
California (mid- and late-winter; diam. 3-1/8-in	1 avocado	284	74	370	5	37	7	17	5	13	22	1.3	630	.24	.43	3.5	30
Florida (late summer, fall; diam. 3-5/8-in	1 avocado	454	78	390	4	33	7	15	4	27	30	1.8	880	.33	.61	4.9	43
Bananas, raw, medium size[e]	1 banana	175	76	100	1	Trace	—	—	—	26	10	.8	230	.06	.07	.8	12
Banana flakes	1 cup	100	3	340	4	1	—	—	—	89	32	2.8	760	.18	.24	2.8	7
Blackberries, raw	1 cup	144	84	85	2	1	—	—	—	19	46	1.3	290	.05	.06	.5	30
Blueberries, raw	1 cup	140	83	85	1	1	—	—	—	21	21	1.4	140	.04	.08	.6	20
Cantaloupes, raw; medium, 5-in diam., about 1 2/3 lbs[e]	1/2 melon	385	91	60	1	Trace	—	—	—	14	27	.8	6,540[i]	.08	.06	1.2	63
Cherries, canned, red, sour, pitted, water pack	1 cup	244	88	105	2	Trace	—	—	—	26	37	.7	1,660	.07	.05	.5	12
Cranberry juice cocktail, canned	1 cup	250	83	165	Trace	Trace	—	—	—	42	13	.8	Trace	.03	.03	.1	40[j]
Cranberry sauce, sweetened, canned, strained	1 cup	277	62	405	Trace	1	—	—	—	104	17	.6	60	.03	.03	.1	6
Dates, pitted, cut	1 cup	178	22	490	4	1	—	—	—	130	105	5.3	90	.16	.17	3.9	0
Figs, dried, large, 2 by 1 in	1 fig	21	23	60	1	Trace	—	—	—	15	26	.6	20	.02	.02	.1	0
Fruit cocktail, canned, in heavy syrup	1 cup	256	80	195	1	Trace	—	—	—	50	23	1.0	360	.05	.03	1.3	5
Grapefruit:																	
Raw, medium, 3 3/4-in diam[e]																	
White	1/2 grapefruit	241	89	45	1	Trace	—	—	—	12	19	.5	10	.05	.02	.2	44
Pink or red	1/2 grapefruit	241	89	50	1	Trace	—	—	—	13	20	.5	540	.05	.02	.2	44
Canned, syrup pack	1 cup	254	81	180	2	Trace	—	—	—	45	33	.8	30	.08	.05	.5	76

	Measure	Grams	Water (%)	Food energy	Protein	Fat				Carbohydrate	Calcium	Iron	k	Thiamin	Riboflavin	Niacin	Ascorbic acid
Grapefruit juice:																	
Fresh	1 cup	246	90	95	1	Trace	—	—	—	23	22	.5	[k]	.09	.04	.4	92
Canned, white:																		
Unsweetened	1 cup	247	89	100	1	Trace	—	—	—	24	20	1.0	20	.07	.04	.4	84
Sweetened	1 cup	250	86	130	1	Trace	—	—	—	32	20	1.0	20	.07	.04	.4	78
Frozen, concentrate, unsweetened:																		
Undiluted, can, 6 fl oz	1 can	207	62	300	4	1	—	—	—	72	70	.8	60	.29	.12	1.4	286
Diluted with 3 parts water, by volume	1 cup	247	89	100	1	Trace	—	—	—	24	25	.2	20	.10	.04	.5	96
Dehydrated crystals	4 oz	113	1	410	6	1	—	—	—	102	100	1.2	80	.40	.20	2.0	396
Prepared with water (1 lb yields about 1 gal)	1 cup	247	90	100	1	Trace	—	—	—	24	22	.2	20	.10	.05	.5	91
Grapes, raw:[e]																		
American type (slip skin)	1 cup	153	82	65	1	1	—	—	—	15	15	.4	100	.05	.03	.2	3
European type (adherent skin)	1 cup	160	81	95	1	Trace	—	—	—	25	17	.6	140	.07	.04	.4	6
Grapejuice:																		
Canned or bottled	1 cup	253	83	165	1	Trace	—	—	—	42	28	.8	—	.10	.05	.5	Trace
Frozen concentrate, sweetened:																		
Undiluted, can, 6 fl oz	1 can	216	53	395	1	Trace	—	—	—	100	22	.9	40	.13	.22	1.5	12
Diluted with 3 parts water, by volume	1 cup	250	86	135	1	Trace	—	—	—	33	8	.3	10	.05	.08	.5	—
Grapejuice drink, canned	1 cup	250	86	135	Trace	Trace	—	—	—	35	8	.3	—	.03	.03	.3	—
Lemons, raw, 2-1/8 in. diam. size 165.[e] Used for juice	1 lemon	110	90	20	1	Trace	—	—	—	6	19	.4	10	.03	.01	.1	39
Lemon juice, raw	1 cup	244	91	60	1	Trace	—	—	—	20	17	.5	50	.07	.02	.2	112
Lemonade concentrate:																		
Frozen, 6 fl oz per can	1 can	219	48	430	Trace	Trace	—	—	—	112	9	.4	40	.04	.07	.7	66
Diluted with 4⅓ parts water, by volume	1 cup	248	88	110	Trace	Trace	—	—	—	28	2	Trace	Trace	Trace	.02	.2	17

[e]Measure and weight apply to entire vegetable or fruit including parts not usually eaten.

[i]Value for varieties with orange-colored flesh; value for varieties with green flesh would be about 540 I.U.

[j]Value listed is based on product with label stating 30 milligrams per 6 fl oz serving.

[k]For white-fleshed varieties value is about 20 I.U. per cup; for red-fleshed varieties, 1,080 I.U. per cup.

[l]Present only if added by the manufacturer. Refer to the label for this information.

FRUITS AND FRUIT PRODUCTS—Con.

Food, Approximate Measure, and Weight (in Grams)		Water (%)	Food Energy (kcal)	Protein (g)	Fat (g)	Fatty Acids			Carbohydrate (g)	Calcium (mg)	Iron (mg)	Vitamin A value (I.U.)	Thiamin (mg)	Riboflavin (mg)	Niacin (mg)	Ascorbic acid (mg)
						Saturated (total) (g)	Unsaturated Oleic (g)	Unsaturated Linoleic (g)								
Lime juice:																
Fresh	1 cup	246	90	65	1	Trace	—	—	—	22	22	.5	20	.05	.02	.2	79
Canned, unsweetened	1 cup	246	90	65	1	Trace	—	—	—	22	22	.5	20	.05	.02	.2	52
Limeade concentrate,frozen:																
Undiluted, can, 6 fl oz	1 can	218	50	410	Trace	Trace	—	—	—	108	11	.2	Trace	.02	.02	.2	26
Diluted with 4⅓ parts water by volume	1 cup	247	90	100	Trace	Trace	—	—	—	27	2	Trace	Trace	Trace	Trace	Trace	5
Oranges, raw 2-5/8 in diam., all commercial varieties[e]	1 orange	180	86	65	1	Trace	—	—	—	16	54	.5	260	.13	.05	.5	66
Orange juice, fresh, all varieties	1 cup	248	88	110	2	1	—	—	—	26	27	.5	500	.22	.07	1.0	124
Canned, unsweetened	1 cup	249	87	120	2	Trace	—	—	—	28	25	1.0	500	.17	.05	.7	100
Frozen concentrate:																
Undiluted, can, 6 fl oz	1 can	213	55	360	5	Trace	—	—	—	87	75	.9	1620	.68	.11	2.8	360
Diluted with 3 parts water by volume	1 cup	249	87	120	2	Trace	—	—	—	29	25	.2	550	.22	.02	1.0	120
Dehydrated crystals	4 oz	113	1	430	6	2	—	—	—	100	95	1.9	1900	.76	.24	3.3	408
Prepared with water (1 lb yields about 1 gal)	1 cup	248	88	115	2	1	—	—	—	27	25	.5	500	.20	.07	1.0	109
Orange-apricot juice drink	1 cup	249	87	125	1	Trace	—	—	—	32	12	.2	1440	.05	.02	.5	40[j]
Orange and grapefruit juice: Frozen concentrate:																
Undiluted, can, 6 fl oz	1 can	210	59	330	4	1	—	—	—	78	61	.8	800	.48	.06	2.3	302
Diluted with 3 parts water by volume	1 cup	248	88	110	1	Trace	—	—	—	26	20	.2	270	.16	.02	.8	102
Papayas, raw, ½-in cubes	1 cup	182	89	70	1	Trace	—	—	—	18	36	.5	3190	.07	.08	.5	102
Peaches: Raw:																
Whole, medium, 2-in diam., about 4 per lb[e]	1 peach	114	89	35	1	Trace	—	—	—	10	9	.5	1320[m]	.02	.05	1.0	7
Sliced	1 cup	168	89	65	1	Trace	—	—	—	16	15	.8	2230[m]	.03	.08	1.6	12

Canned, yellow-fleshed, solids and liquid:																
Syrup pack, heavy:																
Halves or slices	1 cup	257	79	200	1	Trace	—	—	52	10	.8	1100	.02	.06	1.4	7
Water pack	1 cup	245	91	75	1	Trace	—	—	20	10	.7	1100	.02	.06	1.4	7
Dried, uncooked	1 cup	160	25	420	5	1	—	—	109	77	9.6	6240	.02	.31	8.5	28
Cooked, unsweetened, 10-12 halves and juice	1 cup	270	77	220	3	1	—	—	58	41	5.1	3290	.01	.15	4.2	6
Frozen:																
Carton, 12 oz, not thawed	1 carton	340	76	300	1	Trace	—	—	77	14	.7	2210	.03	.14	2.4	135[n]
Pears:																
Raw, 3 by 2½-in diam.[e]	1 pear	182	83	100	1	1	—	—	25	13	.5	30	.04	.07	.2	7
Canned, solids and liquid:																
Syrup pack, heavy:																
Halves or slices	1 cup	255	80	195	1	1	—	—	50	13	.5	Trace	.03	.05	.3	4
Pineapple:																
Raw, diced	1 cup	140	85	75	1	Trace	—	—	19	24	.7	100	.12	.04	.3	24
Canned, heavy syrup pack, solids and liquid:																
Crushed	1 cup	260	80	195	1	Trace	—	—	50	29	.8	120	.20	.06	.5	17
Sliced, slices and juice	2 small or 1 large	122	80	90	Trace	Trace	—	—	24	13	.4	50	.09	.03	.2	8
Pineapple juice, canned	1 cup	249	86	135	1	Trace	—	—	34	37	.7	120	.12	.04	.5	22[h]
Plums, all except prunes:																
Raw, 2-in diam., about 2 oz[e]	1 plum	60	87	25	Trace	Trace	—	—	7	7	.3	140	.02	.02	.3	3
Canned, syrup pack (Italian prunes):																
Plums (with pits) and juice[e]	1 cup	256	77	205	1	Trace	—	—	53	22	2.2	2970	.05	.05	.9	4
Prunes, dried, "softenized," medium:																
Uncooked[e]	4 prunes	32	28	70	1	Trace	—	—	18	14	1.1	440	.02	.04	.4	1
Cooked, unsweetened, 17-18 prunes and ⅓ cup liquid[e]	1 cup	270	66	295	2	1	—	—	78	60	4.5	1860	.08	.18	1.7	2

[e]Measure and weight apply to entire vegetable or fruit including parts not usually eaten.

[h]This is the amount from the fruit. Additional ascorbic acid may be added by the manufacturer. Refer to the label for this information.

[j]Value listed is based on product with label stating 30 milligrams per 6 fl oz serving.

[m]Based on yellow-fleshed varieties; for white-fleshed varieties value is about 50 I.U. per 114 gram peach and 80 I.U. per cup of sliced peaches.

[n]This value includes ascorbic acid added by manufacturer.

Food	Measure	Weight (g)	Water (%)	Food energy	Protein	Fat	Saturated fatty acids	Oleic	Linoleic	Carbohydrate	Calcium	Iron	Vitamin A	Thiamin	Riboflavin	Niacin	Ascorbic acid
Biscuits, baking powder from home recipe with enriched flour, 2-in diam.	1 biscuit	28	27	105	2	5	1	2	1	13	34	.4	Trace	.06	.06	.1	Trace
Biscuits, baking powder from mix, 2-in diam.	1 biscuit	28	28	90	2	3	1	1	1	15	19	.6	Trace	.08	.07	.6	Trace
Bran flakes (40% bran), added thiamin and iron	1 cup	35	3	105	4	1	—	—	—	28	25	12.3	0	.14	.06	2.2	0
Bran flakes with raisins, added thiamin and iron	1 cup	50	7	145	4	1	—	—	—	40	28	13.5	Trace	.16	.07	2.7	0
Breads:																	
Boston brown bread, slice 3 by ¾-in	1 slice	48	45	100	3	1	—	—	—	22	43	.9	0	.05	.03	.6	0
Cracked-wheat bread:																	
Loaf, 1 lb	1 loaf	454	35	1190	40	10	2	5	2	236	399	5.0	Trace	.53	.41	5.9	Trace
Slice, 18 slices per loaf	1 slice	25	35	65	2	1	—	1	—	13	22	.3	Trace	.03	.02	.3	Trace
French or Vienna bread:																	
Enriched, 1 lb loaf	1 loaf	454	31	1315	41	14	3	8	2	251	195	10.0	Trace	1.27	1.00	11.3	Trace
Unenriched, 1 lb loaf	1 loaf	454	31	1315	41	14	3	8	2	251	195	3.2	Trace	.36	.36	3.6	Trace
Italian bread:																	
Enriched, 1 lb loaf	1 loaf	454	32	1250	41	4	Trace	1	2	256	77	10.0	0	1.32	.91	11.8	0
Unenriched, 1 lb loaf	1 loaf	454	32	1250	41	4	Trace	1	2	256	77	3.2	0	.41	.27	3.6	0
Raisin bread:																	
Loaf, 1 lb	1 loaf	454	35	1190	30	13	3	8	2	243	322	5.9	Trace	.23	.41	3.2	Trace
Slice, 18 slices per loaf	1 slice	25	35	65	2	1	—	1	—	13	18	.3	Trace	.01	.02	.2	Trace
Rye bread:																	
American, light (⅓ rye, ⅔ wheat):																	
Loaf, 1 lb	1 loaf	454	36	1100	41	5	—	—	—	236	340	7.3	0	.82	.32	6.4	0
Slice, 18 slices per loaf	1 slice	25	36	60	2	Trace	—	—	—	13	19	.4	0	.05	.02	.4	0
Pumpernickel, loaf, 1 lb	1 loaf	454	34	1115	41	5	—	—	—	241	381	10.9	0	1.04	.64	5.4	0
White bread, enriched:[o]																	
Soft-crumb type:																	
Loaf, 1 lb	1 loaf	454	36	1225	39	15	3	8	2	229	381	11.3	Trace	1.13	.95	10.9	Trace
Slice, 18 slices per loaf	1 slice	25	36	70	2	1	—	—	—	13	21	.6	Trace	.06	.05	.6	Trace
Slice, toasted	1 slice	22	25	70	2	1	—	—	—	13	21	.6	Trace	.06	.05	.6	Trace

[e]Measure and weight apply to entire vegetable or fruit including parts not usually eaten.

[h]This is the amount from the fruit. Additional ascorbic acid may be added by the manufacturer. Refer to the label for this information.

[o]Values for iron, thiamin, riboflavin, and niacin per pound of unenriched white bread would be as follows: soft crumb—Iron - 3.2 mg, Thiamin - .31 mg, Riboflavin - .39 mg, Niacin - 5.0 mg.

Food, Approximate Measure, and Weight (in Grams)		Water (%)	Food Energy (kcal)	Protein (g)	Fat (g)	Fatty Acids Saturated (total) (g)	Unsaturated Oleic (g)	Linoleic (g)	Carbohydrate (g)	Calcium (mg)	Iron (mg)	Vitamin A value (I.U.)	Thiamin (mg)	Riboflavin (mg)	Niacin (mg)	Ascorbic acid (mg)
FRUITS AND FRUIT PRODUCTS—Con.																
Prune juice, canned or bottled	1 cup	256	80	200	1	Trace	—	—	—	49	36	10.5	—	.03	.03	1.0	5[h]
Raisins, seedless:																
Packaged, ½ oz or 1½ tbsp per pkg	1 pkg	14	18	40	Trace	Trace	—	—	—	11	9	.5	Trace	.02	.01	.1	Trace
Cup, pressed down	1 cup	165	18	480	4	Trace	—	—	—	128	102	5.8	30	.18	.13	.8	2
Raspberries, red:																
Raw	1 cup	123	84	70	1	1	—	—	—	17	27	1.1	160	.04	.11	1.1	31
Frozen, 10-oz carton, not thawed	1 carton	284	74	275	2	1	—	—	—	70	37	1.7	200	.06	.17	1.7	59
Rhubarb, cooked, sugar added	1 cup	272	63	385	1	Trace	—	—	—	98	212	1.6	220	.06	.15	.7	17
Strawberries:																
Raw, capped	1 cup	149	90	55	1	1	—	—	—	13	31	1.5	90	.04	.10	1.0	88
Frozen, 10-oz carton, not thawed	1 carton	284	71	310	1	1	—	—	—	79	40	2.0	90	.06	.17	1.5	150
Tangerines, raw, medium, 2-3/8-in diam., size 176[e]	1 tangerine	116	87	40	1	Trace	—	—	—	10	34	.3	360	.05	.02	.1	27
Tangerine juice, canned, sweetened	1 cup	249	87	125	1	1	—	—	—	30	45	.5	1050	.15	.05	.2	55
Watermelon, raw, wedge, 4 by 8 in (1/16 of 10 by 16-in melon, about 2 lbs with rind)[e]	1 wedge	925	93	115	2	1	—	—	—	27	30	2.1	2510	.13	.13	.7	30
GRAIN PRODUCTS																
Bagel, 3-in diam.:																
Egg	1 bagel	55	32	165	6	2	—	—	—	28	9	1.2	30	.14	.10	1.2	0
Water	1 bagel	55	29	165	6	2	—	—	1	30	8	1.2	0	.15	.11	1.4	0
Barley, pearled, light, uncooked	1 cup	200	11	700	16	2	Trace	1	1	158	32	4.0	0	.24	.10	6.2	0

Food, Approximate Measure, and Weight (in Grams)		Water (%)	Food Energy (kcal)	Protein (g)	Fat (g)	Fatty Acids Saturated (total) (g)	Unsaturated Oleic (g)	Linoleic (g)	Carbohydrate (g)	Calcium (mg)	Iron (mg)	Vitamin A value (I.U.)	Thiamin (mg)	Riboflavin (mg)	Niacin (mg)	Ascorbic acid (mg)
GRAIN PRODUCTS—Con.																
White bread, enriched,° soft-crumb type:																
Slice, 22 slices per loaf	1 slice	36	55	2	1	—	—	—	10	17	.5	Trace	.05	.04	.5	Trace
Slice, toasted	1 slice	25	55	2	1	—	—	—	10	17	.5	Trace	.05	.04	.5	Trace
Loaf, 1½ lb	1 loaf	36	1835	59	22	5	12	3	343	571	17.0	Trace	1.70	1.43	16.3	Trace
Slice, 24 slices per loaf	1 slice	36	75	2	1	—	—	—	14	24	.7	Trace	.07	.06	.7	Trace
Slice, toasted	1 slice	25	75	2	1	—	—	—	14	24	.7	Trace	.07	.06	.7	Trace
Slice, 28 slices per loaf	1 slice	36	65	2	1	—	—	—	12	20	.6	Trace	.06	.05	.6	Trace
Slice, toasted	1 slice	25	65	2	1	—	—	—	12	20	.6	Trace	.06	.05	.6	Trace
White bread, enriched,° firm-crumb type:																
Loaf, 1 lb	1 loaf	35	1245	41	17	4	10	2	228	435	11.3	Trace	1.22	.91	10.9	Trace
Slice, 20 slices per loaf	1 slice	35	65	2	1	—	—	—	12	22	.6	Trace	.06	.05	.6	Trace
Slice, toasted	1 slice	24	65	2	1	—	—	—	12	22	.6	Trace	.06	.05	.6	Trace
Loaf, 2 lb	1 loaf	35	2495	82	34	8	20	4	455	871	22.7	Trace	2.45	1.81	21.8	Trace
Slice, 34 slices per loaf	1 slice	35	75	2	1	—	—	—	14	26	.7	Trace	.07	.05	.6	Trace
Slice, toasted	1 slice	35	75	2	1	—	—	—	14	26	.7	Trace	.07	.05	.6	Trace
Whole-wheat bread, soft-crumb type:																
Loaf, 1 lb	1 loaf	36	1095	41	12	2	6	2	224	381	13.6	Trace	1.36	.45	12.7	Trace
Slice, 16 slices per loaf	1 slice	36	65	3	1	—	—	—	14	24	.8	Trace	.09	.03	.8	Trace
Slice, toasted	1 slice	24	65	3	1	—	—	—	14	24	.8	Trace	.09	.03	.8	Trace
Whole-wheat bread, firm-crumb type:																
Loaf, 1 lb	1 loaf	36	1100	48	14	3	6	3	216	449	13.6	Trace	1.18	.54	12.7	Trace
Slice, 18 slices per loaf	1 slice	36	60	3	1	—	—	—	12	25	.8	Trace	.06	.03	.7	Trace
Slice, toasted	1 slice	24	60	3	1	—	—	—	12	25	.8	Trace	.06	.03	.7	Trace
Breadcrumbs, dry, grated	1 cup	6	390	13	5	1	2	1	73	122	3.6	Trace	.22	.30	3.5	Trace
Buckwheat flour, light, sifted	1 cup	12	340	6	1	—	—	—	78	11	1.0	0	.08	.04	.4	0
Bulgur, canned, seasoned	1 cup	56	245	8	4	—	—	—	44	27	1.9	0	.08	.05	4.1	0
Cakes made from cake mixes:																
Angelfood:																
Whole cake	1 cake	34	1645	36	1	—	—	—	377	603	1.9	0	.03	.70	.6	0
Piece, 1/12 of 10-in diam. cake	1 piece	34	135	3	Trace	—	—	—	32	50	.2	0	Trace	.06	.1	0

Food	Measure	g															
Cupcakes, small, 2½-in diam.:																	
Without icing	1 cupcake	25	26	90	1	3	1	1	1	14	40	.1	40	.01	.03	.1	Trace
With chocolate icing	1 cupcake	36	22	130	2	5	2	2	1	21	47	.3	60	.01	.04	.1	Trace
Devil's food, 2-layer, with chocolate icing:																	
Whole cake	1 cake	1107	24	3755	49	136	54	58	16	645	653	8.9	1660	.33	.89	3.3	1
Piece, 1/16 of 9-in diam.	1 piece	69	24	235	3	9	3	4	1	40	41	.6	100	.02	.06	.2	Trace
Cupcake, small, 2½-in diam.	1 cupcake	35	24	120	2	4	1	2	Trace	20	21	.3	50	.01	.03	.1	Trace
Gingerbread:																	
Whole cake	1 cake	570	37	1575	18	39	10	19	9	291	513	9.1	Trace	.17	.51	4.6	2
Piece, 1/9 of 8-in square cake	1 piece	63	37	175	2	4	1	2	1	32	57	1.0	Trace	.02	.06	.5	Trace
White, 2-layer, with chocolate icing:																	
Whole cake	1 cake	1140	21	4000	45	122	45	54	17	716	1129	5.7	680	.23	.91	2.3	2
Piece, 1/16 of 9-in diam. cake	1 piece	71	21	250	3	8	3	3	1	45	70	.4	40	.01	.06	.1	Trace
Cakes made from home recipes:[b]																	
Boston cream pie; piece 1/12 of 8-in diam.	1 piece	69	35	210	4	6	2	3	1	34	46	.3	140	.02	.08	.1	Trace
Fruitcake, dark, made with enriched flour:																	
Loaf, 1-lb	1 loaf	454	18	1720	22	69	15	37	13	271	327	11.8	540	.59	.64	3.6	2
Slice, 1/30 of 8-in loaf	1 slice	15	18	55	1	2	Trace	1	Trace	9	11	.4	20	.02	.1	Trace	
Plain sheet cake:																	
Without icing:																	
Whole cake	1 cake	777	25	2830	35	108	30	52	21	434	497	3.1	1320	.16	.70	1.6	2
Piece, 1/9 of 9-in square cake	1 piece	86	25	315	4	12	3	6	2	48	55	.3	150	.02	.08	.2	Trace
With boiled white icing, piece, 1/9 of 9-in square cake	1 piece	114	23	400	6	12	3	6	2	71	56	.3	150	.02	.08	.2	Trace

[a]Values for iron, thiamin, riboflavin, and niacin per pound of unenriched white bread would be as follows:

	Iron (mg)	Thiamin (mg)	Riboflavin (mg)	Niacin (mg)
Soft crumb	3.2	.31	.39	5.0
Firm crumb	3.2	.32	.59	4.1

[b]Unenriched cake flour used unless otherwise specified.

Food, Approximate Measure, and Weight (in Grams)		Water (%)	Food Energy (kcal)	Protein (g)	Fat (g)	Fatty Acids Saturated (total) (g)	Unsaturated Oleic (g)	Unsaturated Linoleic (g)	Carbohydrate (g)	Calcium (mg)	Iron (mg)	Vitamin A value (I.U.)	Thiamin (mg)	Riboflavin (mg)	Niacin (mg)	Ascorbic acid (mg)
GRAIN PRODUCTS—Con.																
Cakes made from home recipes:p																
Pound:																
Loaf, 8½ by 3½ by 3 in	1 loaf	514	17	2430	29	152	34	68	17	242	108	4.1	1440	.15	.46	1.0	0
Slice, ½-in thick	1 slice	30	17	140	2	9	2	4	1	14	6	.2	80	.01	.03	.1	0
Sponge:																
Whole cake	1 cake	790	32	2345	60	45	14	20	4	427	237	9.5	3560	.40	1.11	1.6	Trace
Piece, 1/12 of 10-in diam. cake	1 piece	66	32	195	5	4	1	2	Trace	36	20	.8	300	.03	.09	.1	Trace
Yellow, 2-layer, without icing:																
Whole cake	1 cake	870	24	3160	39	111	31	53	22	506	618	3.5	1310	.17	.70	1.7	2
Piece, 1/16 of 9-in diam. cake	1 piece	54	24	200	2	7	2	3	1	32	39	.2	80	.01	.04	.1	Trace
Yellow, 2-layer, with chocolate icing:																
Whole cake	1 cake	1203	21	4390	51	156	55	69	23	727	818	7.2	1920	.24	.96	2.4	Trace
Piece, 1/16 of 9-in diam. cake	1 piece	75	21	275	3	10	3	4	1	45	51	.5	120	.02	.06	.2	Trace
Cake icings. See Sugars, Sweets.																
Cookies:																
Brownies with nuts:																
Made from home recipe with enriched flour	1 brownie	20	10	95	1	6	1	3	1	10	8	.4	40	.04	.02	.1	Trace
Made from mix	1 brownie	20	11	85	1	4	1	2	1	13	9	.4	20	.03	.02	.1	Trace
Chocolate chip:																
Made from home recipe with enriched flour	1 cookie	10	3	50	1	3	1	1	1	6	4	.2	10	.01	.01	.1	Trace
Commercial	1 cookie	10	3	50	1	2	1	1	Trace	7	4	.2	10	Trace	Trace	Trace	Trace
Fig bars, commercial	1 cookie	14	14	50	1	1	—	—	Trace	11	11	.2	20	Trace	.01	.1	Trace
Sandwich, chocolate or vanilla, commercial	1 cookie	10	2	50	1	2	1	1	Trace	7	2	.1	0	Trace	Trace	.1	0

Food	Measure	Weight (g)	Food energy (cal)	Protein (g)	Fat (g)	Saturated (g)	Oleic (g)	Linoleic (g)	Carbohydrate (g)	Calcium (mg)	Iron (mg)	Vitamin A (IU)	Thiamin (mg)	Riboflavin (mg)	Niacin (mg)	Ascorbic acid (mg)
Corn flakes, added nutrients:																
Plain	1 cup	25	100	2	Trace	—	—	—	21	4	.4	0	.11	.02	.5	0
Sugar-covered	1 cup	40	155	2	Trace	—	—	—	36	5	.4	0	.16	.02	.8	0
Corn (hominy) grits, degermed, cooked:																
Enriched	1 cup	245	125	3	Trace	—	—	—	27	2	.7	150[q]	.10	.07	1.0	0
Unenriched	1 cup	245	125	3	Trace	—	—	—	27	2	.2	150[q]	.05	.02	.5	0
Cornmeal:																
Whole-ground, unbolted, dry	1 cup	122	435	11	5	1	2	2	90	24	2.9	620[q]	.46	.13	2.4	0
Bolted (nearly whole-grain) dry	1 cup	122	440	11	4	Trace	1	2	91	21	2.2	590[q]	.37	.10	2.3	0
Degermed, enriched:																
Dry form	1 cup	138	500	11	2	—	—	—	108	8	4.0	610[q]	.61	.36	4.8	0
Cooked	1 cup	240	120	3	1	—	—	—	26	2	1.0	140[q]	.14	.10	1.2	0
Degermed, unenriched:																
Dry form	1 cup	138	500	11	2	—	—	—	108	8	1.5	610[q]	.19	.07	1.4	0
Cooked	1 cup	240	120	3	1	—	—	—	26	2	.5	140[q]	.05	.02	.2	0
Corn muffins, made with enriched degermed cornmeal and enriched flour; muffin 2-3/8-in diam.	1 muffin	40	125	3	4	2	2	Trace	19	42	.7	120[q]	.08	.09	.6	Trace
Corn muffins, made with mix, egg, and milk; muffin 2-3/8-in diam.	1 muffin	40	130	3	4	1	2	1	20	96	.6	100	.07	.08	.6	Trace
Corn, puffed, presweetened, added nutrients	1 cup	30	115	2	Trace	—	—	—	27	3	.5	0	.13	.05	.6	0
Corn, shredded, added nutrients	1 cup	25	100	2	Trace	—	—	—	22	1	.6	0	.11	.05	.5	0
Crackers:																
Graham, 2½-in square	4 crackers	28	110	2	3	—	—	—	21	11	.4	0	.01	.06	.4	0
Saltines	4 crackers	11	50	1	1	—	—	1	8	2	.1	0	Trace	Trace	.1	0
Danish pastry, plain (without fruit or nuts):																
Packaged ring, 12 oz	1 ring	340	1435	25	80	24	37	15	155	170	3.1	1050	.24	.51	2.7	Trace
Round piece, approx. 4¼-in diam. by 1 in	1 pastry	65	275	5	15	5	7	3	30	33	.6	200	.05	.10	.5	Trace
Ounce	1 oz	28	120	2	7	2	3	1	13	14	.3	90	.02	.04	.2	Trace

[p] Unenriched cake flour used unless otherwise specified.

[q] This value is based on product made from yellow varieties of corn; white varieties contain only a trace.

Food, Approximate Measure, and Weight (in Grams)		(g)	Water (%)	Food Energy (kcal)	Protein (g)	Fat (g)	Fatty Acids Saturated (total) (g)	Unsaturated Oleic (g)	Unsaturated Lin- oleic (g)	Carbo- hy- drate (g)	Cal- cium (mg)	Iron (mg)	Vita- min A value (I.U.)	Thia- min (mg)	Ribo- flavin (mg)	Niacin (mg)	Ascor- bic acid (mg)
GRAIN PRODUCTS—Con.																	
Doughnuts, cake type	1 doughnut	32	24	125	1	6	1	4	Trace	16	13	.4^r	30	.05^r	.05^r	.4^r	Trace
Farina, quick-cooking, enriched, cooked	1 cup	245	89	105	3	Trace	—	—	—	22	147	.7^s	0	.12^s	.07^s	1.0^s	0
Macaroni, cooked: Enriched:																	
Cooked, firm stage (undergoes additional cooking in a food mixture)	1 cup	130	64	190	6	1	—	—	—	39	14	1.4^s	0	.23^s	.14^s	1.8^s	0
Cooked until tender	1 cup	140	72	155	5	1	—	—	—	32	8	1.3^s	0	.20^s	.11^s	1.5^s	0
Unenriched:																	
Cooked, firm stage (undergoes additional cooking in a food mixture)	1 cup	130	64	190	6	1	—	—	—	39	14	.7	0	.03	.03	.5	0
Cooked until tender	1 cup	140	72	155	5	1	—	—	—	32	11	.6	0	.01	.01	.4	0
Macaroni (enriched) and cheese, baked	1 cup	200	58	430	17	22	10	9	2	40	362	1.8	860	.20	.40	1.8	Trace
Canned	1 cup	240	80	230	9	10	4	3	1	26	199	1.0	260	.12	.24	1.0	Trace
Muffins, with enriched white flour; muffin, 3-in diam.	1 muffin	40	38	120	3	4	1	2	1	17	42	.6	40	.07	.09	.6	Trace
Noodles (egg noodles), cooked:																	
Enriched	1 cup	160	70	200	7	2	1	1	Trace	37	16	1.4^s	110	.22^s	.13^s	1.9^s	0
Unenriched	1 cup	160	70	200	7	2	1	1	Trace	37	16	1.0	110	.05	.03	.6	0
Oats (with or without corn) puffed, added nutrients	1 cup	25	3	100	3	1	—	—	—	19	44	1.2	0	.24	.04	.5	0
Oatmeal or rolled oats, cooked	1 cup	240	87	130	5	2	—	—	1	23	22	1.4	0	.19	.05	.2	0
Pancakes, 4-in diam.: Wheat, enriched flour (home recipe)	1 cake	27	50	60	2	2	Trace	1	Trace	9	27	.4	30	.05	.06	.4	Trace

Buckwheat (made from mix with egg and milk)	1 cake	27	58	55	2	2	1	1	Trace	6	59	.4	60	.03	.04	.2	Trace
Plain or buttermilk (made from mix with egg and milk)	1 cake	27	51	60	2	2	1	1	Trace	9	58	.3	70	.04	.06	.2	Trace
Pie (piecrust made with unenriched flour): Sector, 4-in, 1/7 of 9-in diam. pie:																	
Apple (2-crust)	1 sector	135	48	350	3	15	4	7	3	51	11	.4	40	.03	.03	.5	1
Butterscotch (1-crust)	1 sector	130	45	350	6	14	5	6	2	50	98	1.2	340	.04	.13	.3	Trace
Cherry (2-crust)	1 sector	135	47	350	4	15	4	7	3	52	19	.4	590	.03	.03	.7	Trace
Custard (1-crust)	1 sector	130	58	285	8	14	5	6	2	30	125	.8	300	.07	.21	.4	0
Lemon meringue (1-crust)	1 sector	120	47	305	4	12	4	6	2	45	17	.6	200	.04	.10	.2	4
Mince (2-crust)	1 sector	135	43	365	3	16	4	8	3	56	38	1.4	Trace	.09	.05	.5	1
Pecan (1-crust)	1 sector	118	20	490	6	27	4	16	5	60	55	3.3	190	.19	.08	.4	Trace
Pineapple chiffon (1-crust)	1 sector	93	41	265	6	11	3	5	2	36	22	.8	320	.04	.08	.4	1
Pumpkin (1-crust)	1 sector	130	59	275	5	15	5	6	2	32	66	.7	3210	.04	.13	.7	Trace
Piecrust, baked shell for pie made with:																	
Enriched flour	1 shell	180	15	900	11	60	16	28	12	79	25	3.1	0	.36	.25	3.2	0
Unenriched flour	1 shell	180	15	900	11	60	16	28	12	79	25	.9	0	.05	.05	.9	0
Piecrust mix including stick form:																	
Package, 10-oz, for double crust	1 pkg	284	9	1480	20	93	23	46	21	141	131	1.4	0	.11	.11	2.0	0
Pizza (cheese) 5½-in sector;	1 sector	75	45	185	7	6	2	3	Trace	27	107	.7	290	.04	.12	.7	4
Popcorn, popped:																	
Plain, large kernel	1 cup	6	4	25	1	Trace	—	—	—	5	1	.2	—	—	.01	.1	0
With oil and salt	1 cup	9	3	40	1	2	1	Trace	Trace	5	1	.2	—	—	.01	.2	0
Sugar coated	1 cup	35	4	135	2	1	—	—	—	30	2	.5	—	—	.02	.4	0
Pretzels:																	
Dutch, twisted	1 pretzel	16	5	60	2	1	—	—	—	12	4	.2	0	Trace	Trace	.1	0
Thin, twisted	1 pretzel	6	5	25	1	Trace	—	—	—	5	1	.1	0	Trace	Trace	Trace	0
Stick, small, 2¼-in	10 sticks	3	5	10	Trace	Trace	—	—	—	2	1	Trace	0	Trace	Trace	Trace	0
Stick, regular, 3-1/8-in	5 sticks	3	5	10	Trace	Trace	—	—	—	2	1	Trace	0	Trace	Trace	Trace	0

[r]Based on product made with enriched flour. With unenriched flour, approximate values per doughnut are: Iron, 0.2 milligram; thiamin, 0.01 milligram; riboflavin, 0.03 milligram; niacin, 0.2 milligram.

[s]Iron, thiamin, riboflavin, and niacin are based on the minimum levels of enrichment specified in standards of identity promulgated under the Federal Food, Drug, and Cosmetic Act.

Food, Approximate Measure, and Weight (in Grams)		Water (%)	Food Energy (kcal)	Protein (g)	Fat (g)	Fatty Acids Saturated (total) (g)	Unsaturated Oleic (g)	Unsaturated Linoleic (g)	Carbohydrate (g)	Calcium (mg)	Iron (mg)	Vitamin A value (I.U.)	Thiamin (mg)	Riboflavin (mg)	Niacin (mg)	Ascorbic acid (mg)
GRAIN PRODUCTS—Con.																
Rice, white:																
Enriched:																
Raw	1 cup 185	12	670	12	1	—	—	—	149	44	5.4t	0	.81t	.06t	6.5t	0
Cooked	1 cup 205	73	225	4	Trace	—	—	—	50	21	1.8t	0	.23t	.02t	2.1t	0
Instant, ready-to-serve	1 cup 165	73	180	4	Trace	—	—	—	40	5	1.3t	0	.21t	0	1.7t	0
Unenriched, cooked	1 cup 205	73	225	4	Trace	—	—	—	50	21	.4	0	.04	.02	.8	0
Parboiled, cooked	1 cup 175	73	185	4	Trace	—	—	—	41	33	1.4t	0	.19t	—t	2.1t	0
Rice, puffed, added nutrients	1 cup 15	4	60	1	Trace	—	—	—	13	3	.3	0	.07	.01	.7	0
Rolls, enriched:																
Cloverleaf or pan:																
Home recipe	1 roll 35	26	120	3	3	1	1	1	20	16	.7	30	.09	.09	.8	Trace
Commercial	1 roll 28	31	85	2	2	Trace	1	Trace	15	21	.5	Trace	.08	.05	.6	Trace
Frankfurter or hamburger	1 roll 40	31	120	3	2	1	1	1	21	30	.8	Trace	.11	.07	.9	Trace
Hard, round or rectangular	1 roll 50	25	155	5	2	Trace	1	Trace	30	24	1.2	Trace	.13	.12	1.4	Trace
Rye wafers, whole-grain, 1-7/8 by 3½-in	2 wafers 13	6	45	2	Trace	—	—	—	10	7	.5	0	.04	.03	.2	0
Spaghetti, cooked, tender stage, enriched	1 cup 140	72	155	5	1	—	—	—	32	11	1.3s	0	.20s	.11s	1.5s	0
Spaghetti with meat balls, and tomato sauce:																
Home recipe	1 cup 248	70	330	19	12	4	6	1	39	124	3.7	1590	.25	.30	4.0	22
Canned	1 cup 250	78	260	12	10	2	3	4	28	53	3.3	1000	.15	.18	2.3	5
Spaghetti in tomato sauce with cheese:																
Home recipe	1 cup 250	77	260	9	9	2	5	1	37	80	2.3	1080	.25	.18	2.3	13
Canned	1 cup 250	80	190	6	2	1	1	1	38	40	2.8	930	.35	.28	4.5	10
Waffles, with enriched flour, 7-in diam.	1 waffle 75	41	210	7	7	2	4	1	28	85	1.3	250	.13	.19	1.0	Trace

s Iron, thiamin, riboflavin, and niacin are based on the minimum levels of enrichment specified in standards of identity promulgated under the Federal Food, Drug, and Cosmetic Act.

t Iron, thiamin, and niacin are based on the minimum levels of enrichment specified in standards of identity promulgated under the Federal Food, Drug, and Cosmetic Act. Riboflavin is based on unenriched rice. When the minimum level of enrichment for riboflavin specified in the standards of identity becomes effective the value will be 0.12 milligram per cup of parboiled rice and of white rice.

Waffles, made from mix, enriched, egg and milk added, 7-in diam.	1 waffle	75	42	205	7	8	3	3	1	27	179	1.0	170	.11	.17	.7	Trace
Wheat, puffed, added nutrients	1 cup	15	3	55	2	Trace	—	—	—	12	4	.6	0	.08	.03	1.2	0
Wheat, shredded, plain	1 biscuit	25	7	90	2	1	—	—	—	20	11	.9	0	.06	.03	1.1	0
Wheat flakes, added nutrients	1 cup	30	4	105	3	Trace	—	—	—	24	12	1.3	0	.19	.04	1.5	0
Wheat flours:																	
Whole-wheat, from hard wheats, stirred	1 cup	120	12	400	16	2	Trace	1	1	85	49	4.0	0	.66	.14	5.2	0
All-purpose or family flour, enriched:																	
Sifted	1 cup	115	12	420	12	1	—	—	—	88	18	3.3^s	0	.51^s	.30^s	4.0^s	0
Unsifted	1 cup	125	12	455	13	1	—	—	—	95	20	3.6^s	0	.55^s	.33^s	4.4^s	0
Self-rising, enriched	1 cup	125	12	440	12	1	—	—	—	93	331	3.6^s	0	.55^s	.33^s	4.4^s	0
Cake or pastry flour, sifted	1 cup	96	12	350	7	1	—	—	—	76	16	.5	0	.03	.03	.7	0
FATS, OILS																	
Butter:																	
Regular, 4 sticks per lb:																	
Stick	½ cup	113	16	810	1	92	51	30	3	1	23	0	3750^u	—	—	—	0
Tablespoon (approx. 1/8 stick)	1 tbsp	14	16	100	Trace	12	6	4	Trace	Trace	3	0	470^u	—	—	—	0
Pat (1-in sq. ⅓-in high; 90 per lb)	1 pat	5	16	35	Trace	4	2	1	Trace	Trace	1	0	170^u	—	—	—	0
Whipped, 6 sticks or 2 8-oz containers per lb																	
Stick	½ cup	76	16	540	1	61	34	20	2	Trace	15	0	2500^u	—	—	—	0
Tablespoon (approx. 1/8 stick)	1 tbsp	9	16	65	Trace	8	4	3	Trace	Trace	2	0	310^u	—	—	—	0
Pat (1¼-in sq ⅓-in high; 120 per lb)	1 pat	4	16	25	Trace	3	2	1	Trace	Trace	1	0	130^u	—	—	—	0

^{s}Iron, thiamin, riboflavin, and niacin are based on the minimum levels of enrichment specified in standards of identity promulgated under the Federal Food, Drug, and Cosmetic Act.

^{t}Iron, thiamin, and niacin are based on the minimum levels of enrichment specified in standards of identity promulgated under the Federal Food, Drug, and Cosmetic Act. Riboflavin is based on unenriched rice. When the minimum level of enrichment for riboflavin specified in the standards of identity becomes effective the value will be 0.12 milligram per cup of parboiled rice and of white rice.

^{u}Year-round average.

Food, Approximate Measure, and Weight (in Grams)	Water (%)	Food Energy (kcal)	Protein (g)	Fat (g)	Fatty Acids Saturated (total) (g)	Unsaturated Oleic (g)	Unsaturated Lin-oleic (g)	Carbohydrate (g)	Calcium (mg)	Iron (mg)	Vitamin A value (I.U.)	Thiamin (mg)	Riboflavin (mg)	Niacin (mg)	Ascorbic acid (mg)
FATS, OILS—Con.															
Fats, cooking:															
Lard 1 cup 205	0	1850	0	205	78	94	20	0	0	0	0	0	0	0	0
1 tbsp 13	0	115	0	13	5	6	1	0	0	0	0	0	0	0	0
Vegetable fats 1 cup 200	0	1770	0	200	50	100	44	0	0	0	—	0	0	0	0
1 tbsp 13	0	110	0	13	3	6	3	0	0	0	—	0	0	0	0
Margarine:															
Regular, 4 sticks per lb:															
Stick ½ cup 113	16	815	1	92	17	46	25	1	23	0	3750[V]	—	—	—	0
Tablespoon (approx. 1/8 stick) 1 tbsp 14	16	100	Trace	12	2	6	3	Trace	3	0	470[V]	—	—	—	0
Pat (1-in sq 1/3-in high; 90 per lb) 1 pat 5	16	35	Trace	4	1	2	1	Trace	1	0	170[V]	—	—	—	0
Whipped, 6 sticks per lb:															
Stick ½ cup 76	16	545	1	61	11	31	17	Trace	15	0	2500[V]	—	—	—	0
Soft, 2 - 8-oz tubs per lb:															
Tub 1 tub 227	16	1635	1	184	34	68	68	1	45	0	7500[V]	0	0	—	0
Tablespoon 1 tbsp 14	16	100	Trace	11	2	4	4	Trace	3	0	470[V]	—	—	—	0
Oil, salad or cooking:															
Corn 1 cup 220	0	1945	0	220	22	62	117	0	0	0	—	0	0	0	0
1 tbsp 14	0	125	0	14	1	4	7	0	0	0	—	0	0	0	0
Cottonseed 1 cup 220	0	1945	0	220	55	46	110	0	0	0	—	0	0	0	0
1 tbsp 14	0	125	0	14	4	3	7	0	0	0	—	0	0	0	0
Olive 1 cup 220	0	1945	0	220	24	167	15	0	0	0	—	0	0	0	0
1 tbsp 14	0	125	0	14	2	11	1	0	0	0	—	0	0	0	0
Peanut 1 cup 220	0	1945	0	220	40	103	64	0	0	0	—	0	0	0	0
1 tbsp 14	0	125	0	14	3	7	4	0	0	0	—	0	0	0	0
Safflower 1 cup 220	0	1945	0	220	18	37	165	0	0	0	—	0	0	0	0
1 tbsp 14	0	125	0	14	1	2	10	0	0	0	—	0	0	0	0
Soybean 1 cup 220	0	1945	0	220	33	44	114	0	0	0	—	0	0	0	0
1 tbsp 14	0	125	0	14	2	3	7	0	0	0	—	0	0	0	0

FATS, OILS—Con.

Salad dressings:																
Blue cheese	1 tbsp	15	75	1	8	2	2	4	1	12	Trace	30	Trace	.02	Trace	Trace
Commercial, mayonnaise type:																
Regular	1 tbsp	15	65	Trace	6	1	1	3	2	2	Trace	30	Trace	Trace	Trace	Trace
Special dietary, low-calorie	1 tbsp	16	20	Trace	2	Trace	Trace	1	1	3	Trace	40	Trace	Trace	Trace	—
French:																
Regular	1 tbsp	16	65	Trace	6	1	1	3	3	2	.1	—	—	—	—	—
Special dietary, lowfat with artifical sweeteners	1 tbsp	15	Trace	Trace	Trace	—	—	—	Trace	2	.1	—	—	—	—	—
Home cooked, boiled	1 tbsp	16	25	1	2	1	1	Trace	2	14	.1	80	.01	.03	Trace	Trace
Mayonnaise	1 tbsp	14	100	Trace	11	2	2	6	Trace	3	.1	40	Trace	.01	Trace	—
Thousand island	1 tbsp	16	80	Trace	8	2	2	4	3	2	.1	50	Trace	Trace	Trace	Trace
SUGARS, SWEETS																
Cake icings:																
Chocolate made with milk and table fat	1 cup	275	1035	9	38	21	14	1	185	165	3.3	580	.06	.28	.6	1
Coconut (with boiled icing)	1 cup	166	605	3	13	11	1	Trace	124	10	.8	0	.02	.07	.3	0
Creamy fudge from mix with water only	1 cup	245	830	7	16	5	8	3	183	96	2.7	Trace	.05	.20	.7	Trace
White, boiled	1 cup	94	300	1	0	—	—	—	76	2	Trace	0	Trace	.03	Trace	0
Candy:																
Caramels, plain or chocolate	1 oz	28	115	1	3	2	1	Trace	22	42	.4	Trace	.01	.05	.1	Trace
Chocolate, milk, plain	1 oz	28	145	2	9	5	3	Trace	16	65	.3	80	.02	.10	.1	Trace
Chocolate-coated peanuts	1 oz	28	160	5	12	3	6	2	11	33	.4	Trace	.10	.05	2.1	Trace
Fondant; mints, uncoated; candy corn	1 oz	28	105	Trace	1	—	—	—	25	4	.3	0	Trace	Trace	Trace	0
Fudge, plain	1 oz	28	115	1	4	2	1	Trace	21	22	.3	Trace	.01	.03	.1	Trace
Gum drops	1 oz	28	100	Trace	Trace	—	—	—	25	2	.1	0	0	Trace	Trace	0
Hard	1 oz	28	110	0	Trace	—	—	—	28	6	.5	0	0	0	0	0
Marshmallows	1 oz	28	90	1	Trace	—	—	—	23	5	.5	0	0	Trace	Trace	0
Chocolate-flavored syrup or topping:																
Thin type	1 fl oz	38	90	1	1	Trace	Trace	Trace	24	6	.6	Trace	.01	.03	.2	0
Fudge type	1 fl oz	38	125	2	5	3	2	Trace	20	48	.5	60	.02	.08	.2	Trace

ᵛBased on the average vitamin A content of fortified margarine. Federal specifications for fortified margarine require a minimum of 15,000 I.U. of vitamin A per pound.

Food, Approximate Measure, and Weight (in Grams)		Water (%)	Food Energy (kcal)	Protein (g)	Fat (g)	Fatty Acids Saturated (total) (g)	Unsaturated Oleic (g)	Unsaturated Linoleic (g)	Carbohydrate (g)	Calcium (mg)	Iron (mg)	Vitamin A value (I.U.)	Thiamin (mg)	Riboflavin (mg)	Niacin (mg)	Ascorbic acid (mg)
SUGARS, SWEETS—Con.																
Chocolate-flavored beverage powder (approx. 4 heaping tsp per oz):																
With nonfat dry milk	1 oz	28	2	100	5	1	Trace	Trace	Trace	20	167	.5	10	.04	.21	.2	1
Without nonfat dry milk	1 oz	28	1	100	1	1	Trace	Trace	Trace	25	9	.6	—	.01	.03	.1	0
Honey, strained or extracted	1 tbsp	21	17	65	Trace	0	—	—	—	17	1	.1	Trace	Trace	.01	.1	Trace
Jams and preserves	1 tbsp	20	29	55	Trace	Trace	—	—	—	14	4	.2	Trace	Trace	.01	Trace	Trace
Jellies	1 tbsp	18	29	50	Trace	Trace	—	—	—	13	4	.3	Trace	Trace	.01	Trace	1
Molasses, cane:																
Light (first extraction)	1 tbsp	20	24	50	—	—	—	—	—	13	33	.9	—	.01	.01	Trace	—
Blackstrap (third extraction)	1 tbsp	20	24	45	—	—	—	—	—	11	137	3.2	—	.02	.04	.4	—
Syrups:																
Sorghum	1 tbsp	21	23	55	—	—	—	—	—	14	35	2.6	—	—	.02	Trace	—
Table blends, chiefly corn, light and dark	1 tbsp	21	24	60	0	0	—	—	—	15	9	.8	0	0	0	0	0
Sugars:																
Brown, firm packed	1 cup	220	2	820	0	0	—	—	—	212	187	7.5	0	.02	.07	.4	0
White:																
Granulated	1 cup	200	Trace	770	0	0	—	—	—	199	0	.2	0	0	0	0	0
	1 tbsp	11	Trace	40	0	0	—	—	—	11	0	Trace	0	0	0	0	0
Powdered, stirred before measuring	1 cup	120	Trace	460	0	0	—	—	—	119	0	.1	0	0	0	0	0
MISCELLANEOUS ITEMS																
Barbecue sauce	1 cup	250	81	230	4	17	2	5	9	20	53	2.0	900	.03	.03	.8	13
Beverages, alcoholic:																
Beer	12 fl oz	360	92	150	1	0	—	—	—	14	18	Trace	—	.01	.11	2.2	—
Gin, rum, vodka, whiskey:																
80-proof	1½ fl oz jigger	42	67	100	—	—	—	—	—	Trace	—	—	—	—	—	—	—

86-proof	1½ fl oz jigger	42	64	105	—	—	—	—	Trace	—	—	—	—	—
90-proof	1½ fl oz jigger	42	62	110	—	—	—	—	Trace	—	—	—	—	—
94-proof	1½ fl oz jigger	42	60	115	—	—	—	—	Trace	—	—	—	—	—
100-proof	1½ fl oz jigger	42	58	125	—	—	—	—	Trace	—	—	—	—	—
Wines:														
Dessert	3½ fl oz glass	103	77	140	Trace	0	8	8	—	—	.01	.02	.2	—
Table	3½ fl oz glass	102	86	85	Trace	0	4	9	.4	—	Trace	.01	.1	—
Beverages, carbonated, sweetened, nonalcoholic:														
Carbonated water	12 fl oz	366	92	115	0	0	29	—	—	0	0	0	0	0
Cola type	12 fl oz	369	90	145	0	0	37	—	—	0	0	0	0	0
Fruit-flavored sodas and Tom Collins mixes	12 fl oz	372	88	170	0	0	45	—	—	0	0	0	0	0
Ginger ale	12 fl oz	366	92	115	0	0	29	—	—	0	0	0	0	0
Root beer	12 fl oz	370	90	150	0	0	39	—	—	0	0	0	0	0
Bouillon cubes, approx. ½-in	1 cube	4	4	5	1	Trace	Trace	—	—	—	Trace	—	—	—
Chocolate:														
Bitter or baking	1 oz	28	2	145	3	15	8	22	1.9	20	.01	.07	.4	0
Semisweet, small pieces	1 cup	170	1	860	7	61	97	51	4.4	30	.02	.14	.9	0
Gelatin:														
Plain, dry powder in envelope	1 envelope	7	13	25	6	Trace	0	—	—	—	—	—	—	—
Dessert Powder, 3-oz package	1 pkg	85	2	315	8	0	75	—	—	—	—	—	—	—
Gelatin dessert, prepared with water	1 cup	240	84	140	4	0	34	—	—	—	—	—	—	—
Olives, pickled:														
Green	4 medium or 3 extra large or 2 giant	16	78	15	Trace	2	Trace	8	.2	40	—	—	—	—
Ripe: Mission	3 small or 2 large	10	73	15	Trace	2	Trace	9	.1	10	Trace	Trace	—	—

Food, Approximate Measure, and Weight (in Grams)		Water (%)	Food Energy (kcal)	Protein (g)	Fat (g)	Saturated (total) (g)	Unsaturated Oleic (g)	Unsaturated Linoleic (g)	Carbohydrate (g)	Calcium (mg)	Iron (mg)	Vitamin A value (I.U.)	Thiamin (mg)	Riboflavin (mg)	Niacin (mg)	Ascorbic acid (mg)
MISCELLANEOUS ITEMS—Con.																
Pickles, cucumber:																
Dill, medium, whole, 3¾-in long, 1¼-in diam.	1 pickle	65	93	10	1	Trace	—	—	—	1	17	.7	70	Trace	.01	Trace	4
Fresh, sliced, 1½-in diam., ¼-in thick	2 slices	15	79	10	Trace	Trace	—	—	—	3	5	.3	20	Trace	Trace	Trace	1
Sweet, gherkin, small, whole, approx. 2½-in long, ¾-in diam.	1 pickle	15	61	20	Trace	Trace	—	—	—	6	2	.2	10	Trace	Trace	Trace	1
Relish, finely chopped, sweet	1 tbsp	15	63	20	Trace	Trace	—	—	—	5	3	.1	—	—	—	—	—
Popcorn. See Grain Products.																
Popsicle, 3 fl oz size	1 popsicle	95	80	70	0	0	0	0	0	18	0	Trace	0	0	0	0	0
Pudding, home recipe with starch base:																
Chocolate	1 cup	260	66	385	8	12	7	4	Trace	67	250	1.3	390	.05	.36	.3	1
Vanilla (blanc mange)	1 cup	255	76	285	9	10	5	3	Trace	41	298	Trace	410	.08	.41	.3	2
Pudding mix, dry form, 4 oz package	1 pkg	113	2	410	3	2	1	1	Trace	103	23	1.8	Trace	.02	.08	.5	0
Sherbet	1 cup	193	67	260	2	2	—	—	—	59	31	Trace	120	.02	.06	Trace	4
Soups:																
Canned, condensed, ready-to-serve:																
Prepared with an equal volume of milk:																
Cream of chicken	1 cup	245	85	180	7	10	3	3	3	15	172	.5	610	.05	.27	.7	2
Cream of mushroom	1 cup	245	83	215	7	14	4	4	5	16	191	.5	250	.05	.34	.7	1
Tomato	1 cup	250	84	175	7	7	3	2	1	23	168	.8	1200	.10	.25	1.3	15
Prepared with an equal volume of water:																
Bean with pork	1 cup	250	84	170	8	6	1	2	2	22	63	2.3	650	.13	.08	1.0	3
Beef broth, bouillon consomme	1 cup	240	96	30	5	0	—	—	—	3	Trace	.5	Trace	Trace	.02	1.2	—
Beef noodle	1 cup	240	93	70	4	3	1	1	1	7	7	1.0	50	.05	.07	1.0	Trace

Food	Measure	Grams	Water (%)	Food energy (Cal)	Protein (g)	Fat (g)	Saturated (g)	Oleic (g)	Linoleic (g)	Carbohydrate (g)	Calcium (mg)	Iron (mg)	Vitamin A (IU)	Thiamin (mg)	Riboflavin (mg)	Niacin (mg)	Ascorbic acid (mg)
Clam chowder, Manhattan type (with tomatoes, without milk)	1 cup	245	92	80	2	3	—	—	—	12	34	1.0	880	.02	.02	1.0	—
Cream of chicken	1 cup	240	92	95	3	6	1	2	3	8	24	.5	410	.02	.05	.5	Trace
Cream of mushroom	1 cup	240	90	135	2	10	1	3	5	10	41	.5	70	.02	.12	.7	Trace
Minestrone	1 cup	245	90	105	5	3	—	—	—	14	37	1.0	2350	.07	.05	1.0	—
Split pea	1 cup	245	85	145	9	3	1	2	Trace	21	29	1.5	440	.25	.15	1.5	1
Tomato	1 cup	245	90	90	2	3	Trace	1	1	16	15	.7	1000	.05	.05	1.2	12
Vegetable beef	1 cup	245	92	80	5	2	—	—	—	10	12	.7	2700	.05	.05	1.0	—
Vegetarian	1 cup	245	92	80	2	2	—	—	—	13	20	1.0	2940	.05	.05	1.0	—
Dehydrated, dry form:																	
Chicken noodle (2-oz package)	1 pkg	57	6	220	8	6	2	3	1	33	34	1.4	190	.30	.15	2.4	3
Onion mix (1½-oz package)	1 pkg	43	3	150	6	5	1	2	1	23	42	.6	30	.05	.03	.3	6
Tomato vegetable with noodles (2½-oz pkg)	1 pkg	71	4	245	6	6	2	3	1	45	33	1.4	1700	.21	.13	1.8	18
Frozen, condensed:																	
Clam chowder, New England type (with milk, without tomatoes):																	
Prepared with equal volume of milk	1 cup	245	83	210	9	12	—	—	—	16	240	1.0	250	.07	.29	.5	Trace
Prepared with equal volume of water	1 cup	240	89	130	4	8	—	—	—	11	91	1.0	50	.05	.10	.5	—
Cream of potato:																	
Prepared with equal volume of milk	1 cup	245	83	185	8	10	5	3	Trace	18	208	1.0	590	.10	.27	.5	Trace
Prepared with equal volume of water	1 cup	240	90	105	3	5	3	2	Trace	12	58	1.0	410	.05	.05	.5	—
Cream of shrimp:																	
Prepared with equal volume of milk	1 cup	245	82	245	9	16	—	—	—	15	189	.5	290	.07	.27	.5	Trace
Prepared with equal volume of water	1 cup	240	88	160	5	12	—	—	—	8	38	.5	120	.05	.05	.5	—
Oyster stew:																	
Prepared with equal volume of milk	1 cup	240	83	200	10	12	—	—	—	14	305	1.4	410	.12	.41	.5	Trace
Prepared with equal volume of water	1 cup	240	90	120	6	8	—	—	—	8	158	1.4	240	.07	.19	.5	—

Food, Approximate Measure, and Weight (in Grams)		Water (%)	Food Energy (kcal)	Protein (g)	Fat (g)	Fatty Acids Saturated (total) (g)	Unsaturated Oleic (g)	Lin- oleic (g)	Carbo- hy- drate (g)	Cal- cium (mg)	Iron (mg)	Vita- min A value (I.U.)	Thia- min (mg)	Ribo- flavin (mg)	Niacin (mg)	Ascor- bic acid (mg)
MISCELLANEOUS ITEMS—Con.																
Tapioca, dry quick-cooking	1 cup	152	13	535	1	Trace	—	—	—	131	15	.6	0	0	0	0	0
Tapioca desserts:																
Apple	1 cup	250	70	295	1	Trace	—	—	—	74	8	.5	30	Trace	Trace	Trace	Trace
Cream pudding	1 cup	165	72	220	8	8	4	3	Trace	28	173	.7	480	.07	.30	.2	2
Tartar sauce	1 tbsp	14	34	75	Trace	8	1	1	4	1	3	.1	30	Trace	Trace	Trace	Trace
Vinegar	1 tbsp	15	94	Trace	Trace	0	—	—	—	1	1	.1	—	—	—	—	—
White sauce, medium	1 cup	250	73	405	10	31	16	10	1	22	288	.5	1150	.10	.43	.5	2
Yeast:																
Baker's, dry, active	1 pkg	7	5	20	3	Trace	—	—	—	3	3	1.1	Trace	.16	.38	2.6	Trace
Brewer's, dry	1 tbsp	8	5	25	3	Trace	—	—	—	3	17	1.4	Trace	1.25	.34	3.0	Trace
Yogurt. See Milk, Cheese, Cream, Imitation Cream.																

Appendix *E*

The American College of Sports Medicine Position Statement on Weight Loss in Wrestlers

Despite repeated admonitions by medical, education, and athletic groups ("AMA Committee," 1967; Eriksen, 1967; Kroll, 1967; Rasch & Kroll, 1964; Tipton & Tcheng, 1973) most wrestlers have been inculcated by instruction or accepted tradition to lose weight in order to be certified for a class that is lower than their preseason weight (Tipton & Tcheng, 1970). Studies (Tipton & Tcheng, 1970; Zambraski, Foster, Gross, & Tipton, 1976) of weight losses in high-school and college wrestlers indicate that from 3 to 20% of the preseason body weight is lost before certification or competition occurs. Of this weight loss, most of the decrease occurs in the final days or day before the official weigh-in (Tipton & Tcheng, 1970; Zambraski et al., 1976) with the youngest and/or lightest members of the team losing the highest percentage of their body weight (Tipton & Tcheng, 1970). Under existing rules and practices, it is not uncommon for an individual to repeat this weight losing process many times during the season because successful wrestlers compete in 15 to 30 matches per year *(1975 Program).*

Contrary to existing beliefs, most wrestlers are not "fat" before the season starts (Tipton, 1973). In fact, the fat content of high-school and college wrestlers weighing less than 190 lbs has been shown to range from 1.6 to 15.1% of their body weight with the majority possessing less than 8% (Katch & Michael, 1971; Sinning, 1974; Tcheng & Tipton, 1973). It is well known and documented that wrestlers lose body weight by a combination of food restriction, fluid deprivation, and sweating induced by thermal or exercise procedures (Paul, 1966; Rasch & Kroll, 1964; Tipton & Tcheng, 1970; Zambraski et al., 1976). Of these methods, dehydration through sweating appears to be the method most frequently chosen.

Careful studies on the nature of the weight being lost show that water, fats, and proteins are lost when food restriction and fluid deprivation procedures are followed (Grande, 1961). Moreover, the proportionality between these constituents will change with continued restriction and deprivation. For example, if food restriction is held constant when the volume of fluid being consumed is decreased, more water will be lost from the tissues of the body than before the fluid restriction occurred. The problem becomes more acute when thermal or exercise dehydration occurs because electrolyte losses will accompany the water losses (Kozlowski & Saltin, 1964). Even when 1 to 5 hours are allowed for purposes of rehydration after the weigh-in, this time interval is insufficient for fluid and electrolyte homeostasis to be completely reestablished (Herbert & Ribisl, 1972; Vaccaro, Zauner, & Cade, 1975; Zambraski, Tipton, Tcheng, Jordan, Vailas, & Callahan, 1975; Zambraski et al., 1976).

Since the "making of weight" occurs by combinations of food restriction, fluid deprivation, and dehydration, responsible officials should realize that the single or combined effects of these practices are generally associated with (a) a reduction in muscular strength (Bosco, Terjung, & Greenleaf, 1968; Keys, Brozek, Henschel, Mickelsen, & Taylor, 1950; Taylor, Buskirk, Brozek, Anderson, & Grande, 1957); (b) a decrease in work performance times (Robinson, 1970; Saltin, 1964a, 1964b; Taylor et al., 1957); (c) lower plasma and blood volumes (Costill & Sparks, 1973; Costill, Cote, Miller, Miller, & Wynder, 1975; Robinson, 1970; Saltin, 1964b); (d) a reduction in cardiac functioning during submaximal work conditions which are associated with higher heart rates (Ahlman & Karvonen, 1961; Palmer, 1968; Ribisl & Herbert, 1970; Robinson, 1970; Saltin, 1964b), smaller stroke volumes (Saltin, 1964b), and reduced cardiac outputs (Saltin, 1964b); (e) a lower oxygen consumption, especially with food restriction (Keys et al., 1950; Taylor et al., 1957); (f) an impairment of thermoregulatory processes (Bock, Fox, & Bowers, 1967; Grande, Monagle, Buskirk, & Taylor, 1959; Robinson, 1970); (g) a decrease in renal blood flow (Radigan & Robinson, 1949; Rowell, 1974), and in the volume of fluid being filtered by the kidney (Radigan & Robinson, 1949); (h) a depletion of liver glycogen stores (Hultman & Nilsson, 1973); and (i) an increase in the amount of electrolytes being lost from the body (Costill & Sparks, 1973; Costill et al., 1975; Kozlowski & Saltin, 1964).

Since it is possible for these changes to impede normal growth and development, there is little physiological or medical justification for the use of the weight reduction methods currently followed by many wrestlers. These sentiments have been expressed in part within Rule 1, Section 3, Article 1 of the *Official Wrestling Rule Book* (1975) published by the National Federation of State High School Associations, which states "The Rules Committee recommends that individual state high school associations develop and utilize an effective weight control program which will discourage severe weight reduction and/or wide variations in weight, because this may be harmful to the competitor . . . ." However, until the National Federation of State High School Associations defines the meaning of the terms "severe" and "wide variations," this rule will be ineffective in reducing the abuses associated with the "making of weight."

Therefore, it is the position of the American College of Sports Medicine[1] that the potential health hazards created by the procedures used to "make weight" by wrestlers can be eliminated if state and national organizations will:

1. Assess the body composition of each wrestler several weeks in advance of the competitive season (Clarke, 1974; Katch & Michael, 1971; Sinning, 1974; Tcheng & Tipton, 1973; Wilmore & Behnke, 1969). Individuals with a fat content less than 5% of their certified body weight should receive medical clearance before being allowed to compete.

2. Emphasize the fact that the daily caloric requirements of wrestlers should be obtained from a balanced diet and determined on the basis of age, body surface area, growth and physical activity levels (National Research Council Data, 1965). The minimal caloric needs of wrestlers in high schools and colleges will range from 1,200 to 2,400 kcal/day (Tipton, 1936); therefore, it is the responsibility of coaches, school officials, physicians, and parents to discourage wrestlers from securing less than their minimal needs without prior medical approval.

3. Discourage the practice of fluid deprivation and dehydration. This can be accomplished by:

    a. Educating the coaches and wrestlers on the physiological consequences and medical complications that can occur as a result of these practices.

---

[1]The services of the American College of Sports Medicine are available to assist local and national organizations in implementing these recommendations.

b. Prohibiting the single or combined use of rubber suits, steam rooms, hot boxes, saunas, laxatives, and diuretics to "make weight."

c. Scheduling weigh-ins just prior to competition.

d. Scheduling more official weigh-ins between team matches.

4. Permit more participants per team to compete in those weight classes (119 to 145 lbs) which have the highest percentages of wrestlers certified for competition (Tipton, Tcheng, & Zambraski, 1976).

5. Standardize regulations concerning the eligibility rules at championship tournaments so that individuals can only participate in those weight classes in which they had the highest frequencies of matches throughout the season.

6. Encourage local and county organizations to systematically collect data on the hydration state (Zambraski et al., 1975, 1976) of wrestlers and its relationship to growth and development.

References

Ahlman, K., & Karvonen, M.J. Weight reduction by sweating in wrestlers and its effect on physical fitness. *The Journal of Sports Medicine and Physical Fitness*, 1961, **1**, 58-62.

AMA Committee on the medical aspects of sports, wrestling and weight control. *Journal of the American Medical Association*, 1967, **201**, 541-543.

Bock, W.E., Fox, E.L., & Bowers, R. The effect of acute dehydration upon cardiorespiratory endurance. *The Journal of Sports Medicine and Physical Fitness*, 1967, **7**, 62-72.

Bosco, J.S., Terjung, R.L., & Greenleaf, J.E. Effects of progressive hypohydration on maximal isometric muscular strength. *The Journal of Sports Medicine and Physical Fitness*, 1968, **8**, 81-86.

Clarke, K.S. Predicting certified weight of young wrestlers: A field study of the Tcheng-Tipton method. *Medicine and Science in Sports*, 1974, **6**, 52-57.

Costill, D.L., Cote, R., Miller, E., Miller, T., & Wynder, S. Water and electrolyte replacement during repeated days of work in the heat. *Aviation, Space, and Environmental Medicine*, 1975, **46**, 795-800.

Costill, D.L., & Sparks, K.E. Rapid fluid replacement following thermal dehydration. *Journal of Applied Physiology*, 1973, **34**, 299-303.

Eriksen, F.G. Interscholastic wrestling and weight control: Current plans and their loopholes. *Proceedings of the Eighth National Conference on the Medical Aspects of Sports*, Chicago, AMA, 1967, pp. 34-39.

Grande, F. Nutrition and energy balance in body composition studies. In J. Brozek & A. Henschel (Eds.), *Techniques for measuring body composition*. Washington, DC: National Academy of Sciences and National Research Council, 1961.

Grande, F.J., Monagle, E., Buskirk, E.R., & Taylor, H.L. Body temperature responses to exercise in man on restricted food and water intake. *Journal of Applied Physiology*, 1959, **14**, 194-198.

Herbert, W.G., & Ribisl, P.M. Effects of dehydration upon physical work capacity of wrestlers under competitive conditions. *Research Quarterly*, 1972, **43**, 416-422.

Hultman, E., & Nilsson, L. Liver glycogen as glucose-supplying source during exercise. In J. Keul (Ed.), *Limiting factors of physical performance*. Stuttgart: Georg Thieme, 1973.

1975 Program for the 55th State Wrestling Tournament, Iowa High School Athletic Association, pp. 7-9.

Katch, F.I., & Michael, E.D., Jr. Body composition of high school wrestlers according to age and wrestling weight category. *Medicine and Science in Sports*, 1971, **3**, 190-194.

Keys, A.L., Brozek, J., Henschel, A., Mickelsen, O., & Taylor, H.L. *The biology of human starvation* (Vol. 1). Minneapolis: University of Minnesota Press, 1950.

Kozlowski, S., & Saltin, B. Effect of sweat loss on body fluids. *Journal of Applied Physiology*, 1964, **19**, 1119-1124.

Kroll, W. Guidelines for rules and practices. *Proceedings of the Eighth National Conference on the Medical Aspects of Sports*, Chicago, AMA, 1967, pp. 40-44.

The National Federation 1974-75 wrestling rule book. Elgin, IL: The National Federation Publications.

Palmer, W. Selected physiological responses of normal young men following dehydration and rehydration. *Research Quarterly*, 1968, **39**, 1054-1059.

Paul, W.D. Crash diets in wrestling. *The Journal of the Iowa Medical Society*, 1966, **56**, 835-840.

Radigan, L.R. & Robinson, S. Effect of environmental heat stress and exercise on renal blood flow and filtration rate. *Journal of Applied Physiology*, 1949, **2**, 185-191.

Rasch, P.G., & Kroll, W. *What research tells the coach about wrestling*. Washington: AAHPER, 1964.

Ribisl, P.M., & Herbert, W.G. Effect of rapid weight reduction and subsequent rehydration upon the physical working capacity of wrestlers. *Research Quarterly*, 1970, **41**, 536-541.

Robinson, S. The effect of dehydration on performance. In *Football Injuries*. Washington: National Academy of Science, 1970.

Rowell, L.B. Human cardiovascular adjustments to exercise and thermal stress. *Physiology Reviews*, 1974, **54**, 75-159.

Saltin, B. Aerobic and anaerobic work capacity after dehydration. *Journal of Applied Physiology*, 1964, **19**, 1114-1118. (a)

Saltin, B. Circulatory response to submaximal and maximal exercise after thermal dehydration. *Journal of Applied Physiology*, 1964, **19**, 1125-1132. (b)

Sinning, W.E. Body composition assessment of college wrestlers. *Medicine and Science in Sports*, 1974, **6**, 139-145.

Suggested Daily Dietary Requirement. National Research Council Data. In B.O. Oser, *Hawk's physiological chemistry* (14th ed.). New York: McGraw-Hill, 1965.

Taylor, H.L., Buskirk, E.R., Brozek, J., Anderson, J.T., & Grande, F. Performance capacity and effects of caloric restriction with hard physical work on young men. *Journal of Applied Physiology*, 1957, **10**, 421-429.

Tcheng, T.K., & Tipton, C.M. Iowa wrestling study: Anthropometric measurements and the prediction of a "minimal" body weight for high school wrestlers. *Medicine and Science in Sports*, 1973, **5**, 1-10.

Tipton, C.M. Unpublished calculations on Iowa High School Wrestlers using height and weight surface area nomogram. (Consalazio, C.F., Johnson, R.E., & Pecora, L.J. *Physiological measurements of metabolic functions in man*. New York, McGraw-Hill, 1963, p. 27, which was constructed from the Dubois-Meech formula published in *Archives for Internal Medicine*, 1916, **17**, 863-871), plus the metabolic standards for age used by the Mayo Foundation Standards that were published by Boothby, Berkson, and Dunn in *American Journal of Physiology*, 1936, **116**, 467-484.

Tipton, C.M. Current status of the Iowa Wrestling Study. *The Predicament*, 1973, p.7.

Tipton, C.M., & Tcheng, T.K. Iowa wrestling study: Weight loss in high school students. *Journal of the American Medical Association*, 1970, **214**, 1269-1274.

Tipton, C.M., Tcheng, T.K., & Paul, W.D. Evaluation of the Hall Method for determining minimum wrestling weights. *The Journal of the Iowa Medical Society*, 1969, **59**, 571-574.

Tipton, C.M., Tcheng, T.K., & Zambraski, E.J. Iowa wrestling study: Weight classification systems. *Medicine and Science in Sports*, 1976, **8**, 101-104.

Vaccaro, P., Zauner, C.W., & Cade, J.R. Changes in body weight, hematocrit and plasma protein concentration due to dehydration and rehydration in wrestlers. *Medicine and Science in Sports*, 1975, **7**, 76.

Wilmore, J.H., & Behnke, A. An anthropometric estimation of body density and lean body weight in young men. *Journal of Applied Physiology*, 1969, **27**, 25-31.

Zambraski, E.J., Foster, D.T., Gross, P.M., & Tipton, C.M. Iowa wrestling study: Weight loss and urinary profiles of collegiate wrestlers. *Medicine and Science in Sports*, 1976, **8**, 105-108.

Zambraski, E.J., Tipton, C.M., Tcheng, T.K., Jordan, H.R., Vailas, A.C., & Callahan, A.K. Changes in the urinary profiles of wrestlers prior to and after competition. *Medicine and Science in Sports*, 1975, **7**, 217-220.

Appendix F

The American College of Sports Medicine Position Statement on the Prevention of Heat Injuries During Distance Running

Based on research findings and current rules governing distance running competition, it is the position of the American College of Sports Medicine that:

1. Distance races (> 16 km or 10 miles) should *not* be conducted when the wet bulb temperature—globe temperature[1] exceeds 28 °C (82.4 °F) (Adolph, 1947; Buskirk & Grasley, 1974).

2. During periods of the year, when the daylight dry bulb temperature often exceeds 27° (80°F), distance races should be conducted before 9:00 a.m. or after 4:00 p.m. (Buskirk & Grasley, 1974; Myhre, 1967; Pugh, Corbett, & Johnson, 1957; Wyndham & Strydom, 1969).

3. It is the responsibility of the race sponsors to provide fluids which contain small amounts of sugar (less than 2.5 gram glucose per 100 ml of water) and electrolytes (less than 10 mEq sodium and 5 mEq potassium per liter of solution) (Costill & Saltin, 1974; Fordtran & Saltin, 1967).

From *Medicine and Science in Sports*, 1975, **7**(1), vii. Copyright 1975 by the American College of Sports Medicine. Reprinted with permission.

[1]Adapted from D. Minard, "Prevention of Heat Casualties in the Marine Corps Recruits," *Military Medicine*, 1961, **126**, 261. WB − GT = 0.7(WBT) + 0.2(GT) + 0.1(DBT).

4. Runners should be encouraged to frequently ingest fluids during competition and to consume 400 to 500 ml (13 to 17 oz) of fluid 10 to 15 minutes before competition (Costill & Saltin, 1974; Fordtran & Saltin, 1967; Wyndham & Strydom, 1969).

5. Rules prohibiting the administration of fluids during the first 10 kilometers (6.2 miles) of a marathon race should be amended to permit fluid ingestion at frequent intervals along the race course. In light of the high sweat rates and body temperatures during distance running in the heat, race sponsors should provide "water stations" at 3 to 4 kilometer (2 to 2.5 mile) intervals for all races of 16 kilometers (10 miles) or more (Costill, Kammer, & Fisher, 1970; Pugh et al., 1957; Wyndham & Strydom, 1969).

6. Runners should be instructed in how to recognize the early warning symptoms that precede heat injury. Recognition of symptoms, cessation of running, and proper treatment can prevent heat injury. Early warning symptoms include the following: piloerection on chest and upper arms, chilling, throbbing pressure in the head, unsteadiness, nausea, and dry skin (Buskirk & Grasley, 1974; Wyndham & Strydom, 1969).

7. Race sponsors should make prior arrangements with medical personnel for the care of cases of heat injury. Responsible and informed personnel should supervise each "feeding station." Organizational personnel should reserve the right to stop runners who exhibit clear signs of heat stroke or heat exhaustion.

It is the position of the American College of Sports Medicine that policies established by local, national, and international sponsors of distance running events should adhere to these guidelines. Failure to adhere to these guidelines may jeopardize the health of competitors through heat injury.

Additional Information

The requirements of distance running place great demands on both circulation and body temperature regulation (Costill et al., 1970; Pugh et al., 1957; Wyndham & Strydom, 1969). Numerous studies have reported rectal temperatures in excess of 40.6 °C (105 °F) after races of 6 to 26.2 miles (9.6 to 41.9 kilometers) (Costill et al., 1970; Pugh et al., 1957; Wyndham & Strydom, 1969). Attempting to counterbalance such overheating, runners incur large sweat losses of 0.8 to 1.1 liters/m^2/hr (Costill et al., 1970; Pugh et al., 1957; Wyndham & Strydom, 1969). The resulting body water deficit may total 6 to 10% of the athlete's body weight. Dehydration of these proportions severely limits subsequent sweating, places dangerous demands on circulation, reduces exercise capacity, and exposes the runner to the health hazards associated with hyperthermia (heat stroke, heat exhaustion, and muscle cramps) (Buskirk & Grasley, 1974; Buskirk, Iampietro, & Bass, 1958; Wyndham & Strydom, 1969).

Under moderate thermal conditions, e.g., 65 to 70°F (18.5 to 21.3°C), no cloud cover, relative humidity 49 to 55%, the risk of overheating is still a serious threat to highly motivated distance runners. Nevertheless, distance races are frequently conducted under more severe conditions than these. The air temperature at the 1967 US Pan American Marathon Trial, for example, was 92 to 95°F (33.6 to 35.3°C). Many highly conditioned athletes failed to finish the race and several of the competitors demonstrated overt symptoms of heat stroke (no sweating, shivering, and lack of orientation).

The above consequences are compounded by the current popularity of distance running among middle-aged and aging men and women who may possess significantly less heat tolerance than their younger counterparts. In recent years, races of 10 to 26.2 miles (16 to 41.9 kilometers) have attracted several thousand runners. Since it is likely that distance running enthusiasts will continue to sponsor races under adverse heat conditions, specific steps should be taken to minimize the health threats which accompany such endurance events.

Fluid ingestion during prolonged running (2 hours) has been shown to effectively reduce rectal temperature and minimize dehydration (Costill et al., 1970). Although most competitors consume fluids during races that exceed 1 to 1.5 hours, current international distance running rules prohibit the administration of fluids until the runner has completed 10 miles (16 kilometers). Under such limitations, the competitor is certain to accumulate a large body water deficit (—3%) before any fluids would be ingested. To make the problem more complex, most runners are unable to judge the volume of fluids they consume during competition (Costill et al., 1970). At the 1968 US Olympic Marathon Trial, it was observed that there were body weight losses of 6.1 kg, with an average total fluid ingestion of only 0.14 to 0.35 liter (Costill et al., 1970). It seems obvious that the rules and habits which prohibit fluid administration during distance running preclude any benefits which might be gained from this practice.

Runners who attempt to consume large volumes of sugar solution during competition complain of gastric discomfort (fullness) and an inability to consume fluids after the first few feedings (Costill et al., 1970; Costill & Saltin, 1974; Fordtran & Saltin, 1967). Generally speaking, most runners drink solutions containing 5 to 20 grams of sugar per 100 mililiters of water. Although saline is rapidly emptied from the stomach (25 ml/min), the addition of even small amounts of sugar can drastically impair the rate of gastric emptying (Costill & Saltin, 1974). During exercise in the heat, carbohydrate supplementation is of secondary importance and the sugar content of the oral feedings should be minimized.

References

Adolph, E.F. *Physiology of man in the desert*. New York: Interscience, 1947.

Buskirk, E.R., & Grasley, W.C. Heat injury and conduct of athletes. In W.R. Johnson & E.R. Buskirk (Eds.), *Science and medicine of exercise and sport* (1st ed.) New York: Harper & Row, 1974.

Buskirk, E.R., Iampietro, P.F., & Bass, D.E. Work performance after dehydration: Effects of physical conditioning and heat acclimatization. *Journal of Applied Physiology*, 1958, **12**, 189-194.

Costill, D.L., Kammer, W.F., & Fisher, A. Fluid ingestion during distance running. *Archives of Environmental Health*, 1970, **21**, 520-525.

Costill, D.L., & Saltin, B. Factors limiting gastric emptying during rest and exercise. *Journal of Applied Physiology*, 1974, **37**(5), 679-683.

Fordtran, J.A., & Saltin, B. Gastric emptying and intestinal absorption during prolonged severe exercise. *Journal of Applied Physiology*, 1967, **23**, 331-335.

Myhre, L.G. *Shifts in blood volume during and following acute environmental and work stresses in man*. Unpublished doctoral dissertation, Indiana University, Bloomington, IN, 1967.

Pugh, L.G.C., Corbett, J.I., & Johnson, R.H. Rectal temperatures, weight losses and sweating rates in marathon running. *Journal of Applied Physiology*, 1957, **23**, 347-353.

Wyndham, C.H., & Strydom, N.B. The danger of an inadequate water intake during marathon running. *South African Medical Journal*, 1969, **43**, 893-896.

Appendix G

Charts and Books for Determining the Calories Burned in Various Activities

Activetics, by Charles T. Kuntzleman.
New York: Peter H. Wyden, 1975. ($9.95)
Publisher's address:
Peter H. Wyden
750 Third Ave.
New York, NY 10017

Exercise Equivalents of Foods, by Frank Konishi.
Carbondale, IL: Southern Illinois University Press, 1973. ($4.95)

Pocket Exercise Calorie Counter ($ .95)
Large Exercise Calorie Counter ($2.50)
Publisher's address:
Fitness Finders
178 E. Harmony Rd.
Spring Arbor, MI 49283

Check out your local bookstore.

Activity	kcal/min⁻¹/kg⁻¹	50 / 110	53 / 117	56 / 123	59 / 130	62 / 137	65 / 143	68 / 150	71 / 157	74 / 163	77 / 170	80 / 176	83 / 183	86 / 190	89 / 196	92 / 203	95 / 209	98 / 216
Archery	0.065	3.3	3.4	3.6	3.8	4.0	4.2	4.4	4.6	4.8	5.0	5.2	5.4	5.6	5.8	6.0	6.2	6.4
Badminton	0.097	4.9	5.1	5.4	5.7	6.0	6.3	6.6	6.9	7.2	7.5	7.8	8.1	8.3	8.6	8.9	9.2	9.5
Bakery, general (F)	0.035	1.8	1.9	2.0	2.1	2.2	2.3	2.4	2.5	2.6	2.7	2.8	2.9	3.0	3.1	3.2	3.3	3.4
Basketball	0.138	6.9	7.3	7.7	8.1	8.6	9.0	9.4	9.8	10.2	10.6	11.0	11.5	11.9	12.3	12.7	13.1	13.5
Billiards	0.042	2.1	2.2	2.4	2.5	2.6	2.7	2.9	3.0	3.1	3.2	3.4	3.5	3.6	3.7	3.9	4.0	4.1
Bookbinding	0.038	1.9	2.0	2.1	2.2	2.4	2.5	2.6	2.7	2.8	2.9	3.2	3.2	3.3	3.4	3.5	3.6	3.7
Boxing																		
in ring	0.222	6.9	7.3	7.7	8.1	8.6	9.0	9.4	9.8	10.2	10.6	11.0	11.5	11.9	12.3	12.7	13.1	13.5
sparring	0.138	11.1	11.8	12.4	13.1	13.8	14.4	15.1	15.8	16.4	17.1	17.8	18.4	19.1	19.8	20.4	21.1	21.8
Canoeing																		
leisure	0.044	2.2	2.3	2.5	2.6	2.7	2.9	3.0	3.1	3.3	3.4	3.5	3.7	3.8	3.9	4.0	4.2	4.3
racing	0.103	5.2	5.5	5.8	6.1	6.4	6.7	7.0	7.3	7.6	7.9	8.2	8.5	8.9	9.2	9.5	9.8	10.1
Card playing	0.025	1.3	1.3	1.4	1.5	1.6	1.6	1.7	1.8	1.9	1.9	2.0	2.1	2.2	2.2	2.3	2.4	2.5
Carpentry, general	0.052	2.6	2.8	2.9	3.1	3.2	3.4	3.5	3.7	3.8	4.0	4.2	4.3	4.5	4.6	4.8	4.9	5.1
Carpet sweeping (F)	0.045	2.3	2.4	2.5	2.7	2.8	2.9	3.1	3.2	3.3	3.5	3.6	3.7	3.9	4.0	4.1	4.3	4.4
Carpet sweeping (M)	0.048	2.4	2.5	2.7	2.8	3.0	3.1	3.3	3.4	3.6	3.7	3.8	4.0	4.1	4.3	4.4	4.6	4.7
Circuit-training	0.185	9.3	9.8	10.4	10.9	11.5	12.0	12.6	13.1	13.7	14.2	14.8	15.4	15.9	16.5	17.0	17.6	18.1
Cleaning (F)	0.062	3.1	3.3	3.5	3.7	3.8	4.0	4.2	4.4	4.6	4.8	5.0	5.1	5.3	5.5	5.7	5.9	6.1
Cleaning (M)	0.058	2.9	3.1	3.2	3.4	3.6	3.8	3.9	4.1	4.3	4.5	4.6	4.8	5.0	5.2	5.3	5.5	5.7
Climbing hills																		
with no load	0.121	6.1	6.4	6.8	7.1	7.5	7.9	8.2	8.6	9.0	9.3	9.7	10.0	10.4	10.8	11.1	11.5	11.9
with 5-kg load	0.129	6.5	6.8	7.2	7.6	8.0	8.4	8.8	9.2	9.5	9.9	10.3	10.7	11.1	11.5	11.9	12.3	12.6
with 10-kg load	0.140	7.0	7.4	7.8	8.3	8.7	9.1	9.5	9.9	10.4	10.8	11.2	11.6	12.0	12.5	12.9	13.3	13.7
with 20-kg load	0.147	7.4	7.8	8.2	8.7	9.1	9.6	10.0	10.4	10.9	11.3	11.8	12.2	12.6	13.1	13.5	14.0	14.4
Coal mining																		
drilling coal, rock	0.094	4.7	5.0	5.3	5.5	5.8	6.1	6.4	6.7	7.0	7.2	7.5	7.8	8.1	8.4	8.6	8.9	9.2
erecting supports	0.088	4.4	4.7	4.9	5.2	5.5	5.7	6.0	6.2	6.5	6.8	7.0	7.3	7.6	7.8	8.1	8.4	8.6
shoveling coal	0.108	5.4	5.7	6.0	6.4	6.7	7.0	7.3	7.7	8.0	8.3	8.6	9.0	9.3	9.6	9.9	10.3	10.6
Cooking (F)	0.045	2.3	2.4	2.5	2.7	2.8	2.9	3.1	3.2	3.3	3.5	3.6	3.7	3.9	4.0	4.1	4.3	4.4
Cooking (M)	0.048	2.4	2.5	2.7	2.8	3.0	3.1	3.3	3.4	3.6	3.7	3.8	4.0	4.1	4.3	4.4	4.6	4.7
Cricket																		
batting	0.083	4.2	4.4	4.6	4.9	5.1	5.4	5.6	5.9	6.1	6.4	6.6	6.9	7.1	7.4	7.6	7.9	8.1
bowling	0.090	4.5	4.8	5.0	5.3	5.6	5.9	6.1	6.4	6.7	6.9	7.2	7.5	7.7	8.0	8.3	8.6	8.8

From W.D. McArdle, F.I. Katch, and V.L. Katch, *Exercise Physiology: Energy, Nutrition, and Human Performance.* Philadelphia: Lea & Febiger, 1981. Copyright 1981 by Lea & Febiger. Reprinted with permission.

Activity	kcal/min⁻¹/kg⁻¹	50 / 110	53 / 117	56 / 123	59 / 130	62 / 137	65 / 143	68 / 150	71 / 157	74 / 163	77 / 170	80 / 176	83 / 183	86 / 190	89 / 196	92 / 203	95 / 209	98 / 216
Croquet	0.059	3.0	3.1	3.3	3.5	3.7	3.8	4.0	4.2	4.4	4.5	4.7	4.9	5.1	5.3	5.4	5.6	5.8
Cycling																		
leisure, 5.5 mph	0.064	3.2	3.4	3.6	3.8	4.0	4.2	4.4	4.5	4.7	4.9	5.1	5.3	5.5	5.7	5.9	6.1	6.3
leisure, 9.4 mph	0.100	5.0	5.3	5.6	5.9	6.2	6.5	6.8	7.1	7.4	7.7	8.0	8.3	8.6	8.9	9.2	9.5	9.8
racing	0.169	8.5	9.0	9.5	10.0	10.5	11.0	11.5	12.0	12.5	13.0	13.5	14.0	14.5	15.0	15.5	16.1	16.6
Dancing																		
ballroom	0.051	2.6	2.7	2.9	3.0	3.2	3.3	3.5	3.6	3.8	3.9	4.1	4.2	4.4	4.5	4.7	4.8	5.0
choreographed	0.168	8.4	8.9	9.4	9.9	10.4	10.9	11.4	11.9	12.4	12.9	13.4	13.9	14.4	15.0	15.5	16.0	16.5
"twist," "wiggle"	0.104	5.2	5.5	5.8	6.1	6.4	6.7	7.0	7.3	7.6	7.9	8.2	8.5	8.9	9.2	9.5	9.8	10.1
Digging trenches	0.145	7.3	7.7	8.1	8.6	9.0	9.4	9.9	10.3	10.7	11.2	11.6	12.0	12.5	12.9	13.3	13.8	14.2
Drawing (standing)	0.036	1.8	1.9	2.0	2.1	2.2	2.3	2.4	2.6	2.7	2.8	2.9	3.0	3.1	3.2	3.3	3.4	3.5
Eating (sitting)	0.023	1.2	1.2	1.3	1.4	1.4	1.5	1.6	1.6	1.7	1.8	1.8	1.9	2.0	2.0	2.1	2.2	2.3
Electrical work	0.058	2.9	3.1	3.2	3.4	3.6	3.8	3.9	4.1	4.3	4.5	4.6	4.8	5.0	5.2	5.3	5.5	5.7
Farming																		
barn cleaning	0.135	6.8	7.2	7.6	8.0	8.4	8.8	9.2	9.6	10.0	10.4	10.8	11.2	11.6	12.0	12.4	12.8	13.2
driving harvester	0.040	2.0	2.1	2.2	2.4	2.5	2.6	2.7	2.8	3.0	3.1	3.2	3.3	3.4	3.6	3.7	3.8	3.9
driving tractor	0.037	1.9	2.0	2.1	2.2	2.3	2.4	2.5	2.6	2.7	2.8	3.0	3.1	3.2	3.3	3.4	3.5	3.6
feeding cattle	0.085	4.3	4.5	4.8	5.0	5.3	5.5	5.8	6.0	6.3	6.5	6.8	7.1	7.3	7.6	7.8	8.1	8.3
feeding animals	0.065	3.3	3.4	3.6	3.8	4.0	4.2	4.4	4.6	4.8	5.0	5.2	5.4	5.6	5.8	6.0	6.2	6.4
forking straw bales	0.138	6.9	7.3	7.7	8.1	8.6	9.0	9.4	9.8	10.2	10.6	11.0	11.5	11.9	12.3	12.7	13.1	13.5
milking by hand	0.054	2.7	2.9	3.0	3.2	3.3	3.5	3.7	3.8	4.0	4.2	4.3	4.5	4.6	4.8	5.0	5.1	5.3
milking by machine	0.023	1.2	1.2	1.3	1.4	1.4	1.5	1.6	1.6	1.7	1.8	1.8	1.9	2.0	2.0	2.1	2.2	2.3
shoveling grain	0.085	4.3	4.5	4.8	5.0	5.3	5.5	5.8	6.0	6.3	6.5	6.8	7.1	7.3	7.6	7.8	8.1	8.3
Field hockey	0.134	6.7	7.1	7.5	7.9	8.3	8.7	9.1	9.5	9.9	10.3	10.7	11.1	11.5	11.9	12.3	12.7	13.1
Fishing	0.062	3.1	3.3	3.5	3.7	3.8	4.0	4.2	4.4	4.6	4.8	5.0	5.1	5.3	5.5	5.7	5.9	6.1
Food shopping (F)	0.062	3.1	3.3	3.5	3.7	3.8	4.0	4.2	4.4	4.6	4.8	5.0	5.1	5.3	5.5	5.7	5.9	6.1
Food shopping (M)	0.058	2.9	3.1	3.2	3.4	3.6	3.8	3.9	4.1	4.3	4.5	4.6	4.8	5.0	5.2	5.3	5.5	5.7
Football	0.132	6.6	7.0	7.4	7.8	8.2	8.6	9.0	9.4	9.8	10.2	10.6	11.0	11.4	11.7	12.1	12.5	12.9
Forestry																		
ax chopping, fast	0.297	14.9	15.7	16.6	17.5	18.4	19.3	20.2	21.1	22.0	22.9	23.8	24.7	25.5	26.4	27.3	28.2	29.1
ax chopping, slow	0.085	4.3	4.5	4.8	5.0	5.3	5.5	5.8	6.0	6.3	6.5	6.8	7.1	7.3	7.6	7.8	8.1	8.3
barking trees	0.123	6.2	6.5	6.9	7.3	7.6	8.0	8.4	8.7	9.1	9.5	9.8	10.2	10.6	10.9	11.3	11.7	12.1
carrying logs	0.186	9.3	9.9	10.4	11.0	11.5	12.1	12.6	13.2	13.8	14.3	14.9	15.4	16.0	16.6	17.1	17.7	18.2

Activity	kcal/min⁻¹/kg⁻¹	50 110	53 117	56 123	59 130	62 137	65 143	68 150	71 157	74 163	77 170	80 176	83 183	86 190	89 196	92 203	95 209	98 216
Forestry (Con.)																		
felling trees	0.132	6.6	7.0	7.4	7.8	8.2	8.6	9.0	9.4	9.8	10.2	10.6	11.0	11.4	11.7	12.1	12.5	12.9
hoeing	0.091	4.6	4.8	5.1	5.4	5.6	5.9	6.2	6.5	6.7	7.0	7.3	7.6	7.8	8.1	8.4	8.6	8.9
planting by hand	0.109	5.5	5.8	6.1	6.4	6.8	7.1	7.4	7.7	8.1	8.4	8.7	9.0	9.4	9.7	10.0	10.4	10.7
sawing by hand	0.122	6.1	6.5	6.8	7.2	7.6	7.9	8.3	8.7	9.0	9.4	9.8	10.1	10.5	10.9	11.2	11.6	12.0
sawing, power	0.075	3.8	4.0	4.2	4.4	4.7	4.9	5.1	5.3	5.6	5.8	6.0	6.2	6.5	6.7	6.9	7.1	7.4
stacking firewood	0.088	4.4	4.7	4.9	5.2	5.5	5.7	6.0	6.2	6.5	6.8	7.0	7.3	7.6	7.8	8.1	8.4	8.6
trimming trees	0.129	6.5	6.8	7.2	7.6	8.0	8.4	8.8	9.2	9.5	9.9	10.3	10.7	11.1	11.5	11.9	12.3	12.6
weeding	0.072	3.6	3.8	4.0	4.2	4.5	4.7	4.9	5.1	5.3	5.5	5.8	6.0	6.2	6.4	6.6	6.8	7.1
Furriery	0.083	4.2	4.4	4.6	4.9	5.1	5.4	5.6	5.9	6.1	6.4	6.6	6.9	7.1	7.4	7.6	7.9	8.1
Gardening																		
digging	0.126	6.3	6.7	7.1	7.4	7.8	8.2	8.6	8.9	9.3	9.7	10.1	10.5	10.8	11.2	11.6	12.0	12.3
hedging	0.077	3.9	4.1	4.3	4.5	4.8	5.0	5.2	5.5	5.7	5.9	6.2	6.4	6.6	6.9	7.1	7.3	7.5
mowing	0.112	5.6	5.9	6.3	6.6	6.9	7.3	7.6	8.0	8.3	8.6	9.0	9.3	9.6	10.0	10.3	10.6	11.0
raking	0.054	2.7	2.9	3.0	3.2	3.3	3.5	3.7	3.8	4.0	4.2	4.3	4.5	4.6	4.8	5.0	5.1	5.3
Golf	0.085	4.3	4.5	4.8	5.0	5.3	5.5	5.8	6.0	6.3	6.5	6.8	7.1	7.3	7.6	7.8	8.1	8.3
Gymnastics	0.066	3.3	3.5	3.7	3.9	4.1	4.3	4.5	4.7	4.9	5.1	5.3	5.5	5.7	5.9	6.1	6.3	6.5
Horse-grooming	0.128	6.4	6.8	7.2	7.6	7.9	8.3	8.7	9.1	9.5	9.9	10.2	10.6	11.0	11.4	11.8	12.2	12.5
Horse-racing																		
galloping	0.137	6.9	7.3	7.7	8.1	8.5	8.9	9.3	9.7	10.1	10.6	11.0	11.4	11.8	12.2	12.6	13.0	13.4
trotting	0.110	5.5	5.8	6.2	6.5	6.8	7.2	7.5	7.8	8.1	8.5	8.8	9.1	9.5	9.8	10.1	10.5	10.8
walking	0.041	2.1	2.2	2.3	2.4	2.5	2.7	2.8	2.9	3.0	3.2	3.3	3.4	3.5	3.6	3.8	3.9	4.0
Ironing (F)	0.033	1.7	1.7	1.8	1.9	2.0	2.1	2.2	2.3	2.4	2.5	2.6	2.7	2.8	2.9	3.0	3.1	3.2
Ironing (M)	0.064	3.2	3.4	3.6	3.8	4.0	4.2	4.4	4.5	4.7	4.9	5.1	5.3	5.5	5.7	5.9	6.1	6.3
Judo	0.195	9.8	10.3	10.9	11.5	12.1	12.7	13.3	13.8	14.4	15.0	15.6	16.2	16.8	17.4	17.9	18.5	19.1
Knitting, sewing (F)	0.022	1.1	1.2	1.2	1.3	1.4	1.4	1.5	1.6	1.6	1.7	1.8	1.8	1.9	2.0	2.0	2.1	2.2
Knitting, sewing (M)	0.023	1.2	1.2	1.3	1.4	1.4	1.5	1.6	1.6	1.7	1.8	1.8	1.9	2.0	2.0	2.1	2.2	2.3
Locksmith	0.057	2.9	3.0	3.2	3.4	3.5	3.7	3.9	4.0	4.2	4.4	4.6	4.7	4.9	5.1	5.2	5.4	5.6
Lying at ease	0.022	1.1	1.2	1.2	1.3	1.4	1.4	1.5	1.6	1.6	1.7	1.8	1.8	1.9	2.0	2.0	2.1	2.2
Machine-tooling																		
machining	0.048	2.4	2.5	2.7	2.8	3.0	3.1	3.3	3.4	3.6	3.7	3.8	4.0	4.1	4.3	4.4	4.6	4.7
operating lathe	0.052	2.6	2.8	2.9	3.1	3.2	3.4	3.5	3.7	3.8	4.0	4.2	4.3	4.5	4.6	4.8	4.9	5.1
operating punch press	0.088	4.4	4.7	4.9	5.2	5.5	5.7	6.0	6.2	6.5	6.8	7.0	7.3	7.6	7.8	8.1	8.4	8.6

Activity	kcal·min⁻¹/kg⁻¹	50 / 110	53 / 117	56 / 123	59 / 130	62 / 137	65 / 143	68 / 150	71 / 157	74 / 163	77 / 170	80 / 176	83 / 183	86 / 190	89 / 196	92 / 203	95 / 209	98 / 216
Machine-tooling (Con.)																		
tapping and drilling	0.065	3.3	3.4	3.6	3.8	4.0	4.2	4.4	4.6	4.8	5.0	5.2	5.4	5.6	5.8	6.0	6.2	6.4
welding	0.052	2.6	2.8	2.9	3.1	3.2	3.4	3.5	3.7	3.8	4.0	4.2	4.3	4.5	4.6	4.8	4.9	5.1
working sheet metal	0.048	2.4	2.5	2.7	2.8	3.0	3.1	3.3	3.4	3.6	3.7	3.8	4.0	4.1	4.3	4.4	4.6	4.7
Marching, rapid	0.142	7.1	7.5	8.0	8.4	8.8	9.2	9.7	10.1	10.5	10.9	11.4	11.8	12.2	12.6	13.1	13.5	13.9
Mopping floor (F)	0.062	3.1	3.3	3.5	3.7	3.8	4.0	4.2	4.4	4.6	4.8	5.0	5.1	5.3	5.5	5.7	5.9	6.1
Mopping floor (M)	0.058	2.9	3.1	3.2	3.4	3.6	3.8	3.9	4.1	4.3	4.5	4.6	4.8	5.0	5.2	5.0	5.5	5.7
Music playing																		
accordion (sitting)	0.032	1.6	1.7	1.8	1.9	2.0	2.1	2.2	2.3	2.4	2.5	2.6	2.7	2.8	2.8	2.9	3.0	3.1
cello (sitting)	0.041	2.1	2.2	2.3	2.4	2.5	2.7	2.8	2.9	3.0	3.2	3.3	3.4	3.5	3.6	3.8	3.9	4.0
conducting	0.039	2.0	2.1	2.2	2.3	2.4	2.5	2.7	2.8	2.9	3.0	3.1	3.2	3.4	3.5	3.6	3.7	3.8
drums (sitting)	0.066	3.3	3.5	3.7	3.9	4.1	4.3	4.5	4.7	4.9	5.1	5.3	5.5	5.7	5.9	6.1	6.3	6.6
flute (sitting)	0.035	1.8	1.9	2.0	2.1	2.2	2.3	2.4	2.5	2.6	2.7	2.8	2.9	3.0	3.1	3.2	3.3	3.4
horn (sitting)	0.029	1.5	1.5	1.6	1.7	1.8	1.9	2.0	2.1	2.1	2.2	2.3	2.4	2.5	2.6	2.7	2.8	2.8
organ (sitting)	0.053	2.7	2.8	3.0	3.1	3.3	3.4	3.6	3.8	3.9	4.1	4.2	4.4	4.6	4.7	4.9	5.0	5.2
piano (sitting)	0.040	2.0	2.1	2.2	2.4	2.5	2.6	2.7	2.8	3.0	3.1	3.2	3.3	3.4	3.6	3.7	3.8	3.9
trumpet (standing)	0.031	1.6	1.6	1.7	1.8	1.9	2.0	2.1	2.2	2.3	2.4	2.5	2.6	2.7	2.8	2.9	2.9	3.0
violin (sitting)	0.045	2.3	2.4	2.5	2.7	2.8	2.9	3.1	3.2	3.3	3.5	3.6	3.7	3.9	4.0	4.1	4.3	4.4
woodwind (sitting)	0.032	1.6	1.7	1.8	1.9	2.0	2.1	2.2	2.3	2.4	2.5	2.6	2.7	2.8	2.8	2.9	3.0	3.1
Painting, inside	0.034	1.7	1.8	1.9	2.0	2.1	2.2	2.3	2.4	2.5	2.6	2.7	2.8	2.9	3.0	3.1	3.2	3.3
Painting, outside	0.077	3.9	4.1	4.3	4.5	4.8	5.0	5.2	5.5	5.7	5.9	6.2	6.4	6.6	6.9	7.1	7.3	7.5
Planting seedlings	0.070	3.5	3.7	3.9	4.1	4.3	4.6	4.8	5.0	5.2	5.4	5.6	5.8	6.0	6.2	6.4	6.7	6.9
Plastering	0.078	3.9	4.1	4.4	4.6	4.8	5.1	5.3	5.5	5.8	6.0	6.2	6.5	6.7	6.9	7.2	7.4	7.6
Printing	0.035	1.8	1.9	2.0	2.1	2.2	2.3	2.4	2.5	2.6	2.7	2.8	2.9	3.0	3.1	3.2	3.3	3.4
Running, cross-country	0.163	8.2	8.6	9.1	9.6	10.1	10.6	11.1	11.6	12.1	12.6	13.0	13.5	14.0	14.5	15.0	15.5	16.0
Running, horizontal																		
11 min, 30 s per mile	0.135	6.8	7.2	7.6	8.0	8.4	8.8	9.2	9.6	10.0	10.5	10.9	11.3	11.7	12.1	12.5	12.9	13.3
9 min per mile	0.193	9.7	10.2	10.8	11.4	12.0	12.5	13.1	13.7	14.3	14.9	15.4	16.0	16.6	17.2	17.8	18.3	18.9
8 min per mile	0.208	10.8	11.3	11.9	12.5	13.1	13.6	14.2	14.8	15.4	16.0	16.5	17.1	17.7	18.3	18.9	19.4	20.0
7 min per mile	0.228	12.2	12.7	13.3	13.9	14.5	15.0	15.6	16.2	16.8	17.4	17.9	18.5	19.1	19.7	20.3	20.8	21.4
6 min per mile	0.252	13.9	14.4	15.0	15.6	16.2	16.7	17.3	17.9	18.5	19.1	19.6	20.2	20.8	21.4	22.0	22.5	23.1
5 min, 30 s per mile	0.289	14.5	15.3	16.2	17.1	17.9	18.8	19.7	20.5	21.4	22.3	23.1	24.0	24.9	25.7	26.6	27.5	28.3

Activity	kcal/min⁻¹/kg⁻¹	50 / 110	53 / 117	56 / 123	59 / 130	62 / 137	65 / 143	68 / 150	71 / 157	74 / 163	77 / 170	80 / 176	83 / 183	86 / 190	89 / 196	92 / 203	95 / 209	98 / 216
Scraping paint	0.063	3.2	3.3	3.5	3.7	3.9	4.1	4.3	4.5	4.7	4.9	5.0	5.2	5.4	5.6	5.8	6.0	6.2
Scrubbing floors (F)	0.109	5.5	5.8	6.1	6.4	6.8	7.1	7.4	7.7	8.1	8.4	8.7	9.0	9.4	9.7	10.0	10.4	10.7
Scrubbing floors (M)	0.108	5.4	5.7	6.0	6.4	6.7	7.0	7.3	7.7	8.0	8.3	8.6	9.0	9.3	9.6	9.9	10.3	10.6
Shoe repair, general	0.045	2.3	2.4	2.5	2.7	2.8	2.9	3.1	3.2	3.3	3.5	3.6	3.7	3.9	4.0	4.1	4.3	4.4
Sitting quietly	0.021	1.1	1.1	1.2	1.2	1.3	1.4	1.4	1.5	1.6	1.6	1.7	1.7	1.8	1.9	1.9	2.0	2.1
Skiing, hard snow																		
level, moderate speed	0.119	6.0	6.3	6.7	7.0	7.4	7.7	8.1	8.4	8.8	9.2	9.5	9.9	10.2	10.6	10.9	11.3	11.7
level, walking	0.143	7.2	7.6	8.0	8.4	8.9	9.3	9.7	10.2	10.6	11.0	11.4	11.9	12.3	12.7	13.2	13.6	14.0
uphill, maximum speed	0.274	13.7	14.5	15.3	16.2	17.0	17.8	18.6	19.5	20.3	21.1	21.9	22.7	23.6	24.4	25.2	26.0	26.9
Skiing, soft snow																		
leisure (F)	0.111	4.9	5.2	5.5	5.8	6.1	6.4	6.7	7.0	7.3	7.5	7.8	8.1	8.4	8.7	9.0	9.3	9.6
leisure (M)	0.098	5.6	5.9	6.2	6.5	6.9	7.2	7.5	7.9	8.2	8.5	8.9	9.2	9.5	9.9	10.2	10.5	10.9
Skindiving, as frogman																		
considerable motion	0.276	13.8	14.6	15.5	16.3	17.1	17.9	18.8	19.6	20.4	21.3	22.1	22.9	23.7	24.6	25.4	26.2	27.0
moderate motion	0.206	10.3	10.9	11.5	12.2	12.8	13.4	14.0	14.6	15.2	15.9	16.5	17.1	17.7	18.3	19.0	19.6	20.2
Snowshoeing, soft snow	0.166	8.3	8.8	9.3	9.8	10.3	10.8	11.3	11.8	12.3	12.8	13.3	13.8	14.3	14.8	15.3	15.8	16.3
Squash	0.212	10.6	11.2	11.9	12.5	13.1	13.8	14.4	15.1	15.7	16.3	17.0	17.6	18.2	18.9	19.5	20.1	20.8
Standing quietly (F)	0.025	1.3	1.3	1.4	1.5	1.6	1.6	1.7	1.8	1.9	1.9	2.0	2.1	2.2	2.2	2.3	2.4	2.5
Standing quietly (M)	0.027	1.4	1.4	1.5	1.6	1.7	1.8	1.8	1.9	2.0	2.1	2.2	2.2	2.3	2.4	2.5	2.6	2.6
Steel mill, working in																		
fettling	0.089	4.5	4.7	5.0	5.3	5.5	5.8	6.1	6.3	6.6	6.9	7.1	7.4	7.7	7.9	8.2	8.5	8.7
forging	0.100	5.0	5.3	5.6	5.9	6.2	6.5	6.8	7.1	7.4	7.7	8.0	8.3	8.6	8.9	9.2	9.5	9.8
hand rolling	0.137	6.9	7.3	7.7	8.1	8.5	8.9	9.3	9.7	10.1	10.6	11.0	11.4	11.8	12.2	12.6	13.0	13.4
merchant mill rolling	0.145	7.3	7.7	8.1	8.6	9.0	9.4	9.9	10.3	10.7	11.2	11.6	12.0	12.5	12.9	13.3	13.8	14.2
removing slag	0.178	8.9	9.4	10.0	10.5	11.0	11.6	12.1	12.6	13.2	13.7	14.2	14.8	15.3	15.8	16.4	16.9	17.4
tending furnace	0.126	6.3	6.7	7.1	7.4	7.8	8.2	8.6	8.9	9.3	9.7	10.1	10.5	10.8	11.2	11.6	12.0	12.3
tipping molds	0.092	4.6	4.9	5.2	5.4	5.7	6.0	6.3	6.5	6.8	7.1	7.4	7.6	7.9	8.2	8.5	8.7	9.0
Stock clerking	0.054	2.7	2.9	3.0	3.2	3.3	3.5	3.7	3.8	4.0	4.2	4.3	4.5	4.6	4.8	5.0	5.1	5.3
Swimming																		
backstroke	0.169	8.5	9.0	9.5	10.0	10.5	11.0	11.5	12.0	12.5	13.0	13.5	14.0	14.5	15.0	15.5	16.1	16.6
breast stroke	0.162	8.1	8.6	9.1	9.6	10.0	10.5	11.0	11.5	12.0	12.5	13.0	13.4	13.9	14.4	14.9	15.4	15.9
crawl, fast	0.156	7.8	8.3	8.7	9.2	9.7	10.1	10.6	11.1	11.5	12.0	12.5	12.9	13.4	13.9	14.4	14.8	15.3

Activity	kcal/min⁻¹/kg⁻¹	50 kg / 110 lb	53 / 117	56 / 123	59 / 130	62 / 137	65 / 143	68 / 150	71 / 157	74 / 163	77 / 170	80 / 176	83 / 183	86 / 190	89 / 196	92 / 203	95 / 209	98 / 216
Swimming (Con.)																		
crawl, slow	0.128	6.4	6.8	7.2	7.6	7.9	8.3	8.7	9.1	9.5	9.9	10.2	10.6	11.0	11.4	11.8	12.2	12.5
side stroke	0.122	6.1	6.5	6.8	7.2	7.6	7.9	8.3	8.7	9.0	9.4	9.8	10.1	10.5	10.9	11.2	11.6	12.0
treading, fast	0.170	8.5	9.0	9.5	10.0	10.5	11.1	11.6	12.1	12.6	13.1	13.6	14.1	14.6	15.1	15.6	16.2	16.7
treading, normal	0.062	3.1	3.3	3.5	3.7	3.8	4.0	4.2	4.4	4.6	4.8	5.0	5.1	5.3	5.5	5.7	5.9	6.1
Table tennis	0.068	3.4	3.6	3.8	4.0	4.2	4.4	4.6	4.8	5.0	5.2	5.4	5.6	5.8	6.1	6.3	6.5	6.7
Tailoring																		
cutting	0.041	2.1	2.2	2.3	2.4	2.5	2.7	2.8	2.9	3.0	3.2	3.3	3.4	3.5	3.6	3.8	3.9	4.0
hand-sewing	0.032	1.6	1.7	1.8	1.9	2.0	2.1	2.2	2.3	2.4	2.5	2.6	2.7	2.8	2.8	2.9	3.0	3.1
machine-sewing	0.045	2.3	2.4	2.5	2.7	2.8	2.9	3.1	3.2	3.3	3.5	3.6	3.7	3.9	4.0	4.1	4.3	4.4
pressing	0.062	3.1	3.3	3.5	3.7	3.8	4.0	4.2	4.4	4.6	4.8	5.0	5.1	5.3	5.5	5.7	5.9	6.1
Tennis	0.109	5.5	5.8	6.1	6.4	6.8	7.1	7.4	7.7	8.1	8.4	8.7	9.0	9.4	9.7	10.0	10.4	10.7
Typing																		
electric	0.027	1.4	1.4	1.5	1.6	1.7	1.8	1.8	1.9	2.0	2.1	2.2	2.2	2.3	2.4	2.5	2.6	2.6
manual	0.031	1.6	1.6	1.7	1.7	1.9	2.0	2.1	2.2	2.3	2.4	2.5	2.6	2.7	2.8	2.9	2.9	3.0
Volleyball	0.050	2.5	2.7	2.8	3.0	3.1	3.3	3.4	3.6	3.7	3.9	4.0	4.2	4.3	4.5	4.6	4.8	4.9
Walking, normal pace																		
asphalt road	0.080	4.0	4.2	4.5	4.7	5.0	5.2	5.4	5.7	5.9	6.2	6.4	6.6	6.9	7.1	7.4	7.6	7.8
fields and hillsides	0.082	4.1	4.3	4.6	4.8	5.1	5.3	5.6	5.8	6.1	6.3	6.6	6.8	7.1	7.3	7.5	7.8	8.0
grass track	0.081	4.1	4.3	4.5	4.8	5.0	5.3	5.5	5.8	6.0	6.2	6.5	6.7	7.0	7.2	7.5	7.7	7.9
plowed field	0.077	3.9	4.1	4.3	4.5	4.8	5.0	5.2	5.5	5.7	5.9	6.2	6.4	6.6	6.9	7.1	7.3	7.5
Wallpapering	0.048	2.4	2.5	2.7	2.8	3.0	3.1	3.3	3.4	3.6	3.7	3.8	4.0	4.1	4.3	4.4	4.6	4.7
Watch repairing	0.025	1.3	1.3	1.4	1.5	1.6	1.6	1.7	1.8	1.9	1.9	2.0	2.1	2.2	2.2	2.3	2.4	2.5
Window cleaning (F)	0.059	3.0	3.1	3.3	3.5	3.7	3.8	4.0	4.2	4.4	4.5	4.7	4.9	5.1	5.3	5.4	5.6	5.8
Window cleaning (M)	0.058	2.9	3.1	3.2	3.4	3.6	3.8	3.9	4.1	4.3	4.5	4.6	4.8	5.0	5.2	5.3	5.5	5.7
Writing (sitting)	0.029	1.5	1.5	1.6	1.7	1.8	1.9	2.0	2.1	2.1	2.2	2.3	2.4	2.5	2.6	2.7	2.8	2.8

Data from E.W. Bannister and S.R. Brown, "The relative energy requirements of physical activity," In H.B. Falls, (Ed.), *Exercise Physiology*. New York: Academic Press, 1968; E.T. Howley and M.E. GLover, "The caloric costs of running and walking one mile for men and women," *Medicine and Science in Sports*, 1974, **6**, 235; R. Passmore and J.V.G.A. Durnin, "Human energy expenditure," *Physiological Reviews*, 1955, **35**, 801.

Note. Symbols (M) and (F) denote experiments for males and females, respectively.

Appendix H

Sources on Converting Athletes to Nutritionally Sound Weight Loss and Weight Gain Programs

Food For Sport, by Nathan J. Smith.
Palo Alto, CA: Bull Publishing, 1976. ($6.95)
Publisher's address:
Bull Publishing Company
P.O. Box 208
Palo Alto, CA 94302

Habits, Not Diets: The Real Way to Weight Control,
by James M. Ferguson.
Palo Alto, CA: Bull Publishing, 1976. ($9.95)

How to Convert Kids from What They Eat to What They Oughta,
by Polly Greenberg.
New York: Ballantine Books, 1978. ($2.50)

Nutrition and the Athlete, by J.J. Morella & R.J. Turchetti.
New York: Mason/Charter, 1976. ($6.95)

Nutrition for Athletes.
Washington, DC: AAHPER, 1971. ($2.50)

Appendix *I*

The American College of Sports Medicine Position Statement on the Use and Abuse of Anabolic-Androgenic Steroids in Sports

The Use and Abuse of
Anabolic-Androgenic Steroids in Sports

Based on a comprehensive survey of the world literature and a careful analysis of the claims made for and against the efficacy of anabolic-androgenic steroids in improving human physical performance, it is the position of the American College of Sports Medicine that:

1. The administration of anabolic-androgenic steroids to healthy humans below age 50 in medically approved therapeutic doses often does not of itself bring about any significant improvements in strength, aerobic endurance, lean body mass, or body weight.

2. There is no conclusive scientific evidence that extremely large doses of anabolic-androgenic steroids either aid or hinder athletic performance.

3. The prolonged use of oral anabolic-androgenic steroids

From *Medicine and Science in Sports*, 1977, **9**(4), xi. Copyright 1977 by the American College of Sports Medicine. Reprinted with permission.

(C_{17}—alkylated derivatives of testosterone) has resulted in liver disorders in some persons. Some of these disorders are apparently reversible with the cessation of drug usage, but others are not.

4. The administration of anabolic-androgenic steroids to male humans may result in a decrease in testicular size and function and a decrease in sperm production. Although these effects appear to be reversible when small doses of steroids are used for short periods of time, the reversibility of the effects of large doses over extended periods of time is unclear.

5. Serious and continuing effort should be made to educate male and female athletes, coaches, physical educators, physicians, trainers, and the general public regarding the inconsistent effects of anabolic-androgenic steroids on improvement of human physical performance and the potential dangers of taking certain forms of these substances, especially in large doses, for prolonged periods.

Research Background for the Position Statement

This position stand has been developed from an extensive survey and analysis of the world literature in the fields of medicine, physiology, endocrinology, and physical education. Although the reactions of humans to the use of drugs, including hormones or drugs which simulate the actions of natural hormones, are individual and not entirely predictable, some conclusions can nevertheless be drawn with regard to what desirable and what undesirable effects may be achieved. Accordingly, whereas positive effects of drugs may sometimes arise because persons have been led to expect such changes ("placebo" effect) (Byerly, 1976), repeated experiments of a similar nature often fail to support the initial positive effects and lead to the conclusion that any positive effect that does exist may not be substantial.

1. Administration of testosterone-like synthetic drugs which have anabolic (tissue building) and androgenic (development of male secondary sex characteristics) properties in amounts up to twice those normally prescribed for medical use has been associated with increased strength, lean body mass and/or body weight in some studies (Bowers & Reardon, 1972; Johnson, Fisher, Sylvester, & Hofheins, 1972; Johnson & O'Shea, 1969; O'Shea, 1971; O'Shea & Winkler, 1970; Stanford & Moffett, 1974; Steinbach, 1968; Stromme, Meen, & Aakvaag, 1974) but not in others (Casner, Early, & Carlson, 1971; Fahey & Brown, 1973; Fowler, Gardner, & Egstrom, 1965; Golding, Freydinger, & Fishel, 1974; Johnson, Roundy, Allsen, Fisher, & Sylvester, 1975; Samuels, Henschel, & Kays, 1942; Stromme et al., 1974). One study (Golding et al., 1974) reported an increase in the

amount of weight the steroid group could lift compared to controls but found no difference in isometric strength which suggests a placebo effect in the drug group, a learning effect or possibly a differential drug effect on isotonic compared to isometric strength. An initial report of enhanced aerobic endurance after administration of an anabolic-androgenic steroid (Johnson & O'Shea, 1969) has not been confirmed (Bowers & Reardon, 1972; Casner et al., 1971; Johnson et al., 1975; O'Shea & Winkler, 1970). Because of the lack of adequate control groups in many studies it seems likely that some of the positive effects on strength that have been reported are due to "placebo" effects (Ariel & Saville, 1972; Byerly, 1976), but a few apparently well-designed studies have also shown beneficial effects of steroid administration on muscular strength and lean body mass. Some of the discrepancies in results may also be due to differences in the type of drug administered, the method of drug administration, the nature of the exercise programs involved, the duration of the experiment, and individual differences in sensitivity to the administered drug. High-protein dietary supplements do not insure the effectiveness of the steroids (Golding et al., 1974; Johnson et al., 1975; Stromme et al., 1974). Because of the many failures to show improved muscular strength, lean body mass, or body weight after therapeutic doses of anabolic-androgenic steroids, it is obvious that for many individuals any benefits are likely to be small and not worth the health risks involved.

2. Testimonial evidence by individual athletes suggests that athletes often use much larger doses of steroids than those ordinarily prescribed by physicians and those evaluated in published research. Because of the health risks involved with the long-term use of high doses and requirements for informed consent it is unlikely that scientifically acceptable evidence will be forthcoming to evaluate the effectiveness of such large doses of drugs on athletic performance.

3. Alterations of normal liver function have been found in as many as 80% of one series of 69 patients treated with C_{17}—alkylated testosterone derivatives (oral-anabolic-androgenic steroids) (Sanchez-Medal, Gomez-Leal, Duarte, & Guadalupe-Rico, 1969). Cholestasis has been observed histologically in the livers of persons taking these substances (Sherlock, 1968). These changes appear to be benign and reversible (Shahidi, 1973). Five reports (Bagheri & Boyer, 1974; Burger & Marcuse, 1952; Kantzen & Silny, 1960; Sherlock, 1968; Ziegenfuss & Carabasi, 1973) document the occurrence of peliosis hepatitis in 17 patients without evidence of significant liver disease who were treated with C_{17}—alkylated androgenic steroids. Seven of these patients died of liver failure. The first case of hepato-cellular carcinoma associated with taking an androgenic-anabolic steroid was reported in 1965 (Recant & Lacy, 1965). Since then at least 13 other

patients taking C_{17}—alkylated androgenic steroids have developed hepato-cellular carcinoma (Bernstein, Hunter, & Yachrin, 1971; Farrell, Joshua, Uren, Baird, Perkins, & Kraienberg, 1975; Guy & Auxlander, 1973; Harkness, Kalshaw, & Hobson, 1975; Henderson, Richmond, & Sumerling, 1972; Johnson, 1975; Johnson, Feagler, Lerner, Majems, Siegel, Hartman, & Thomas, 1972; Meadows, Naiman, & Valdes-Dapena, 1974). In some cases dosages as low as 10-15 mg/day taken for only 3 or 4 months have caused liver complications (Golding et al., 1974; Meadows et al., 1974).

4. Administration of therapeutic doses of androgenic-anabolic steroids in men often (Harkness et al., 1975; Kilshaw, Harkness, Hobson, & Smith, 1975) but not always (Aakvaag & Stromme, 1974; Fahey & Brown, 1973; Johnson et al., 1972), reduces the output of testosterone and gonadotropins and reduces spermatogenesis. Some steroids are less potent than others in causing these effects (Aakvaag & Stromme, 1974). Although these effects on the reproductive system appear to be reversible in animals, the long-term results of taking large doses by humans is unknown.

5. Precise information concerning the abuse of anabolic steroids by female athletes is unavailable. Nevertheless, there is no reason to believe females will not be tempted to adopt the use of these medicines. The use of anabolic steroids by females, particularly those who are either prepubertal or have not attained full growth, is especially dangerous. The undesired side effects include masculinization (Allen, Fine, Necheles, & Dameshek, 1968; Sanchez-Medal et al., 1969; Shahidi, 1973), disruption of normal growth pattern (Shahidi, 1973), voice changes (Allen et al., 1968; Shahidi, 1973; Silink & Firkin, 1968), acne (Allen et al., 1968; Sanchez-Medal et al., 1969; Shahidi, 1973; Silink & Firkin, 1968), hirsutism (Sanchez-Medal et al., 1969; Shahidi, 1973; Silink & Firkin, 1968), and enlargement of the clitoris (Sanchez-Medal, 1969). The long-term effects on reproductive function are unknown, but anabolic steroids may be harmful in this area. Their ability to interfere with the menstrual cycle has been well documented (Sanchez-Medal, 1969).

For these reasons, all concerned with advising, training, coaching, and providing medical care for female athletes should exercise all persuasions available to prevent the use of anabolic steroids by female athletes.

References

Aakvaag, A., & Stromme, S.B. The effect of mesterolone administration to normal men on the pituitary-testicular function. *Acta Endocrinologica*, 1974, **77**, 380-386.

Allen, D.M., Fine, M.H., Necheles, T.F., & Dameshek, W. Oxymetholone therapy in aplastic anemia. *Blood*, 1968, **32**, 83-89.

Ariel, G., & Saville, W. Anabolic steroids: The physiological effects of placebos. *Medicine and Science in Sports*, 1972, **4**, 124-126.

Bagheri, S.A., & Boyer, J.L. Peliosis hepatitis associated with androgenic-anabolic steroid therapy. *Annals of Internal Medicine*, 1974, **81**, 610-618.

Bernstein, M.S., Hunter, R.L., & Yachrin, S. Hepatoma and peliosis hepatitis developing in a patient with Fanconi's anemia. *New England Journal of Medicine*, 1971, **284**, 1135-1136.

Bowers, R., & Reardon, J. Effects of methandro-stenolone (Dianabol) on strength development and aerobic capacity. *Medicine and Science in Sports*, 1972, **4**, 54.

Burger, R.A., & Marcuse, P.M. Peliosis hepatitis, report of a case. *American Journal of Clinical Pathology*, 1952, **22**, 569-573.

Byerly, H. Explaining and exploiting placebo effects. *Prospectives in Biology and Medicine*, 1976, **19**, 423-436.

Casner, S. Early, R., & Carlson, B.R. Anabolic steroid effects on body composition in normal young men. *Journal of Sports Medicine and Physical Fitness*, 1971, **11**, 98-103.

Fahey, T.D., & Brown, C.H. The effects of an anabolic steroid on the strength, body composition, and endurance of college males when accompanied by a weight training program. *Medicine and Science in Sports*, 1973, **5**, 272-276.

Farrell, G.C., Joshua, D.E., Uren, R.F., Baird, P.J., Perkins, K.W., & Kraienberg, H. Androgen-induced hepatoma. *Lancet*, 1975, **1**, 430-431.

Fowler, W.M., Jr., Gardner, G.W., & Egstrom, G.H. Effect of an anabolic steroid on physical performance of young men. *Journal of Applied Physiology*, 1965, **20**, 1038-1040.

Golding, L.A., Freydinger, J.E., & Fishel, S.S. Weight, size and strength unchanged by steroids. *The Physician and Sportsmedicine*, 1974, **2**, 39-45.

Guy, J.T., & Auxlander, M.O. Androgenic steroids and hepatocellular carcinoma. *Lancet*, 1973, **1**, 148.

Harkness, R.A., Kalshaw, B.H., & Hobson, B.M. Effects of large doses of anabolic steroids. *British Journal of Sports Medicine*, 1975, **9**, 70-73.

Henderson, J.T., Richmond, J., & Sumerling, M.D. Androgenic-anabolic steroid therapy and hepato-cellular carcinoma. *Lancet*, 1972, **1**, 934.

Johnson, F.L. The association of oral androgenic-anabolic steroids and life threatening disease. *Medicine and Science in Sports*, 1975, **7**, 284-286.

Johnson, F.L., Feagler, J.R., Lerner, K.G., Majems, P.W., Siegel,

M., Hartman, J.R., & Thomas, E.D. Association of androgenic-anabolic steroid therapy with development of hepato-cellular carcinoma. *Lancet*, 1972, **2**, 1273-1276.

Johnson, L.C., Fisher, G., Sylvester, L.J., & Hofheins, C.C. Anabolic steroid: Effects on strength, body weight, O_2 uptake and spermatogenesis in mature males. *Medicine and Science in Sports*, 1972, **4**, 43-45.

Johnson, L.C., & O'Shea, P.P. Anabolic steroid: Effects on strength development. *Science*, 1969, **164**, 957-959.

Johnson, L.C., Roundy, E.S., Allsen, P., Fisher, A.G., & Sylvester, L.J. Effect of anabolic steroid treatment on endurance. *Medicine and Science in Sports*, 1975, **7**, 287-289.

Kantzen, W., & Silny, J. Peliosis hepatitis after administration of fluoxymesterone. *Canadian Medical Association Journal*, 1960, **83**, 860-862.

Kilshaw, B.H., Harkness, R.A., Hobson, B.M., & Smith, A.W.M. The effects of large doses of the anabolic steroid, methandrostenone, on an athlete. *Clinical Endocrinology*, 1975, **4**, 537-541.

Meadows, A.T., Naiman, J.L., & Valdes-Dapena, M.V. Hepatoma associated with androgen therapy for aplastic anemia. *Journal of Pediatrics*, 1974, **84**, 109-110.

McCredie, K.B. Oxymetholone in refractory anaemia. *British Journal of Haematology*, 1969, **17**, 265-273.

O'Shea, J.P. The effects of an anabolic steroid on dynamic strength levels of weight lifters. *Nutritional Reports International*, 1971, **4**, 363-370.

O'Shea, J.P., & Winkler, W. Biochemical and physical effects of an anabolic steroid in competitive swimmers and weight lifters. *Nutritional Reports International*, 1970, **2**, 351-362.

Recant, L., & Lacy, P. Fanconi's anemia and hepatic cirrhosis. Clinicopathologic Conference. *American Journal of Medicine*, 1965, **39**, 464-475.

Samuels, L.T., Henschel, A.F., & Kays, A. Influence of methyltestosterone on muscular work and creatine metabolism in normal young men. *Journal of Clinical Endocrinology and Metabolism*, 1942, **2**, 649-654.

Sanchez-Medal, L., Gomez-Leal, A., Duarte, L., & Guadalupe-Rico, M. Anabolic-androgenic steroids in the treatment of acquired aplastic anemia. *Blood*, 1969, **34**, 283-300.

Shahidi, N.T. Androgens and erythropoiesis. *New England Journal of Medicine*, 1973, **289**, 72-79.

Sherlock, S. *Disease of the liver and biliary system* (4th ed.). Philadelphia: F.A. Davis, 1968.

Silink, J., & Firkin, B.G. An analysis of hypoplastic anaemia with special reference to the use of oxymetholone ("Adroyd") in its therapy. *Australian Annals of Medicine*, 1968, **17**, 224-235.

Stanford, B.A., & Moffat, R. Anabolic steroid: Effectiveness as an ergogenic aid to experienced weight trainers. *The Journal of Sports Medicine and Physical Fitness*, 1974, **14**, 191-197.

Steinbach, M. Uber den Einfluss anabolen Wirkstoffe und Korpergewicht Muskelkraft and Muskeltraining. *Sportarzt und Sportmedizin*, 1968, **11**, 485-492.

Stromme, S.B., Meen, H.D., & Aakvaag, A. Effects of an androgenic-anabolic steroid on strength development and plasma testosterone levels in normal males. *Medicine and Science in Sports*, 1974, **6**, 203-208.

Ward, P. The effect of an anabolic steroid on strength and lean body mass. *Medicine and Science in Sports*, 1973, **5**, 277-282.

Zak, F.G. Peliosis hepatitis. *American Journal of Pathology*, 1950, **26**, 1-15.

Ziegenfuss, J., & Carabasi, R. Androgens and hepato-cellular carcinoma. *Lancet*, 1973, **1**, 262.

Appendix J
Using the Adipometer™

Many of the same instructions presented in chapter 2 on using the skinfold caliper apply to using the Adipometer™ skin caliper available from Ross Laboratories. The skinfolds are taken on the right side of the body. Use considerable care in locating the precise site for the measurement. Once you have located the correct site, firmly grasp the skin between the left (right if you're left-handed) thumb and forefinger and lift up the skin with its underlying fat tissue. Now, take the caliper in hand and place the "jaws" on either side of the skinfold. Place your thumb (index finger if you're left-handed) on the caliper's "trigger lever," which is marked "PRESS." An expensive and accurate caliper will have a built-in spring that exerts a constant tension on the jaws as they close on the skinfold. Because the Adipometer™ has no such spring, you must apply the tension by pressing the caliper together until the short black line on the trigger lever is aligned with the short black line (marked "ALIGN") on the main arm.

When these two lines are aligned, find the indicator line and read the measurement to the nearest millimeter. Release the tension and remove the caliper. Repeat this procedure three times for each skinfold site and record the values. Remember that these values may be somewhat less accurate than those taken with the more expensive caliper, but practice and good judgment will make the Adipometer™ a useful tool in your athletes' weight control program.